For Sarah Lucia
and her perm...
guests,
— Al

The
COUNTRY VET'S

Home
Remedies
for
Cats

David Kay

Consultant: H. Ellen Whiteley, D.V.M.

Publications International, Ltd.

David Kay is a freelance writer who specializes in animal topics. A regular contributor to *The Veterinary Technician*, he also has written for *Cat Fancy, Pet Review, CATS Magazine*, and *The Animals' Agenda*. For 13 years, he served as education director of Tree House Animal Foundation, a Chicago-based humane agency. He has a bachelor of science degree in ecology, ethology, and evolution.

H. Ellen Whiteley, D.V.M., has been a practicing veterinarian for nearly 30 years, with a specialty in small animal medicine. She has headed a small animal clinical relief practice and a veterinary house call service with an emphasis on feline medicine and surgery. In addition to her clinical experience, she is the author of *Understanding and Training Your Cat or Kitten* and has written for *Veterinary Forum, Woman Veterinarian*, and *Veterinary Medicine*.

Illustrations: Brian Jensen
Editorial Assistance: Kelly Boyer Sagert

Cover photo: **Thomas Firak/Photri.**

Louis Weber, C.E.O.
Publications International, Ltd.
7373 North Cicero Avenue
Lincolnwood, Illinois 60646

Permission is never granted for commercial purposes.

Manufactured in China

8 7 6 5 4 3 2 1

ISBN 0-7853-2448-8

Library of Congress Card Catalog Number: 97-69907

CONTENTS

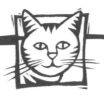

INTRODUCTION

You folks may have heard that cats have nine lives. Well, maybe that's true—and maybe it isn't. But one thing is for sure: The only life that matters to the cat you have right now (or are going to get) is the one she's going to share with you. And that means you ought to take the best possible care of your cat.

Now you might think that there are more than enough "how-to" books around and even more books than that about cats—which means a "how-to" cat book like this one is about as welcome as a hard frost in April. But if you've read this far, you already know that this book is a little different. Say what you'd like about country folk, but you have to agree they have good common sense. "Horse sense" we call it—and I reckon that applies particularly to the country vet.

So this book won't have any ten-dollar names of diseases, parts of the body, or medicines in it. If a country vet talks to you about your cat's ears, that's what he calls them: "ears." That's "ears" and not "pinnae," like they're called in the textbooks. Likewise, he'll give you advice about how to deal with your cat's worms—if she has any. That's "worms" and not "intestinal parasites."

Besides being written in plain English, this book also shares generations of country common sense with you. Over time, people who live close to the earth figure out what works and what doesn't. They understand that if you take the right care of the land and the things that live and grow in, on, and under it, all those things flourish almost without trying. But if you're careless, it can all fade away faster than you can believe. Yes, you might get a few good seasons out of it, but then all of a sudden one spring, nothing seems to be growing anymore.

The same logic applies to your cat. Good food, good habits, and good exercise go a long way to keep your cat flourishing (and you, too, come to think of it) and nip health problems in the bud. But since your cat can't talk and she can't understand that eating cat food is good for her but eating a rubber band isn't, you have to do that work for the both of you. You're not alone, though—this book is here to help you.

Of course, even the best cared-for cat is going to have her share of times when she's feeling under the weather. But paying close attention to the early signs and signals and applying good old country common sense can mean shorter, less severe, or at the very least more tolerable sicknesses. You've just got to know what to look for and what to do. Lucky for you, the country vet knows all about that—and it's all in these pages.

Now before we go any further, I don't want you to think that if you buy this book, you'll never have to spend another dime on the veterinarian. That wouldn't be too smart of me, would it? And I don't just mean that it would be bad business for the country vet. I mean, there are plenty of things that just can't be done at home—and shouldn't be. But there are plenty more things you can do to prevent, treat, and speed up the healing of lots of different medical and behavioral problems your cat might have.

Maybe you already noticed that even though the name of this book is *The Country Vet's Home Remedies for Cats* there's a bit more to be found between these two covers than just remedies. That's because we're talking about cats, here. Cats are living, breathing critters like you and me—not some kind of vending machine with fur where if you put the right things in the right amount in, you get what you want. That's the quarrel I have with some of those big-time specialist city vets I know. They treat a specific problem and don't look at the whole picture.

It's funny, I hear the word "holistic" all the time now. It's supposed to be a newfangled way of doing medicine for people—and animals, too. But that's how country folk have done things for as long as there have been country folk. Every good farmer knows that if your corn yields are going down, you can't just plant more seeds and pile on more fertilizer. You've got to consider weather, erosion, soil conditions—the whole shebang.

I tell you all this as a warning: If you picked up this book because your cat isn't using her litter box and you flipped right to the remedies section, you're doing yourself and your cat a grave disservice. Read the other parts—about care and feeding and behavior—first. Take the time to enjoy this book. Besides learning about a variety of common physical problems, you'll find all kinds of valuable information in this book, from choosing the right cat to making your home safe for your pet. Then take the time to get to know your cat—really know your cat—and you might see a remedy that you won't find in any book.

You see, in a sense, you are the country vet, too. While there's no substitute for regular veterinary care, there's a lot you can do at home to keep your cat healthy and happy. You've got plenty of common sense, and this book will just help you tap into it and put you on the right path to caring for your cat.

One more thing: Be extra sure to read the sections called "When to Call the Vet." *The Country Vet's Home Remedies for Cats* is not meant as a substitute for professional veterinary medical care or advice. The remedies and advice in this book have been checked with practicing veterinarians and animal care experts, but your own vet should be the final authority.

Good health to you and your cat!

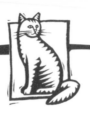

First Steps

I'll confess that my favorite way to while away a summer afternoon is at the minor-league baseball park in the next county. I'm also one of those people who can't really enjoy the game without keeping score. You know the old saying, "You can't tell the players without a scorecard." I have to buy one—along with one of those little pencils—as soon as I walk into the park.

Likewise, to take the best care of your cat you need two essentials right at the start: your own veterinarian and, of course, a cat. This chapter will show you how to find both.

In fact, even if you already have a cat, read on—you never know when you may want to get another one or find a new vet.

MATCH YOUR CAT TO YOUR LIFESTYLE

Before you actually get a cat, figure out what kind of cat you want: kitten or grown-up cat; longhair or shorthair; purebred or alley cat; male or female; tabby, patched, or solid-color.

If you've got your heart set on a particular size, age, sex, breed, or look of cat, do a little extra research before you set out to find one. You might be surprised to find that the look you love doesn't fit well with your lifestyle. For example, if you like a quiet home, a Siamese may not be the cat for you: They're notorious "talkers." Likewise, a Persian is gorgeous to look at, but unless you're committed to do almost daily grooming (or to pay a professional to do it every week or so), a nice shorthair cat might be a better idea. Do you travel a lot? Then you need a more mature cat—at least eight months old or more. Two cats are better still so they can keep each other company while you're away.

CAT OR KITTEN?

Everybody loves kittens. They're cute, funny, and cuddly—there's no doubt about it. But don't make the mistake that they're "babies." By the time a kitten is ready to be away from his mother and live in your home, he can walk, run, jump, and climb like the feline equivalent of a ten-year-old child. What's more, if you get a kitten today, in just a few short months you'll have a full-grown cat—a cat who will live an average of 12 to 15 years.

If you have the time, environment, and energy to raise a kitten, by all means do it—it's a wonderful experience. Just remember that kittens are high-maintenance. They demand a lot of attention. They need routine veterinary care consisting of booster shots, worming, and spaying or neutering. Most all young kittens start off affectionate and passive, but they need some socialization and training to stay that way; and even still, you won't know what their adult personality will be like until they grow up.

Finally, very young children and very young kittens usually don't mix well. It's nice to think that a toddler and a ten-week-old kitten can "grow up together," but it really doesn't happen that way. In six months, that little ball of fur your child could carry around will have grown into ten-pounds-plus of adult cat, and your three-year-old will be . . . three and a half years old!

Finding the Right Cat

"Nobody really owns a cat," my old pal, Hoke Mitchell, likes to say. "You just make a deal with 'em. You agree to open your home and heart, and he agrees to let you have him sleep in your favorite chair and get first dibs on that big old trout you caught this morning."

Well, it's easier to humor old Hoke when he says things like that, so let's just say for the sake of argument (or to avoid one) that he's right. Maybe you can't really own a cat, but the real question is, what's the best way to go about getting one?

There's certainly no danger of a cat shortage in these United States— there are plenty of cats to go around and then some. In most parts of the country, you could just open your front door at sunup, and a cat would probably walk in before you finished breakfast. Heck, there are some city neighborhoods where you can't spit without hitting a stray cat. Not that either one of these activities is recommended, mind you.

In fact, the number of cats around puts you in somewhat of a quandary. How do you choose the right one? Will it be healthy? What about hidden health or behavior problems? What happens to the cat if things don't work out in your home?

Getting a cat isn't like getting a lawn mower or a hair dryer; they don't come with guarantees. Each one is going to be different, which means unique joys and problems come with every cat. Still, sources for cats should help you make a decision. Although the source can't promise the cat will never get sick, they can take steps to give the cat the best possible chances of staying well. Good sources for finding the right cat for you include:

> The smallest breed of domesticated cat is the Singapura, with the average male weighing six pounds and the average female weighing only four pounds.

Friends and neighbors. The odds are somebody you know has a cat or kittens in need of a home. Many times, taking a cat from a neighbor or friend works out best for everyone, especially if it's a kitten from your neighbor's cat's litter or an allergic friend's family pet. Your personal relationship with this source usually means you'll get the straight story on this particular cat, too. A couple of warnings about getting your cat from a friend or neighbor, though: Don't expect the cat to have the extensive veterinary care that a cat from a shelter or breeder has, and be careful about mixing business and friendship.

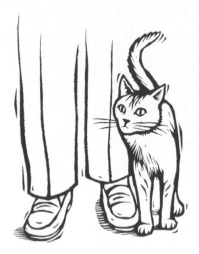

Tales from the Country Vet

Animals seem to know I'm on their side—cats especially. I can't tell you how many times I've been walking along, when out of nowhere comes some tabby, tail up and meowing to beat the band. So when a young black and white shorthair cat approached me out of some tall grass a few years back, I didn't think much of it.

He was a tidy looking young fellow, obviously somebody's pet. When I'd spent the requisite amount of time making a fuss over him, I sent him on his way. "Go on home, now," I told him as I walked away. I made it about six steps, when I nearly tripped over a furry body darting in, out, and around my ankles. "Hey, now," I admonished the little cat kindly. "I said go on home." Determined not to encourage him any more, I set off again at a healthy pace.

Well, I'm sure you know where this story is going. That little guy followed me for more than a mile, right to my front door. I couldn't complain. After all, he had only been following my instructions. I kept telling him to "go home"—and that's just what he did.

First Steps

Animal shelters. Millions of homeless cats end up being euthanized in animal shelters every year. Adopting from a shelter saves a life, makes room for another cat, and is an inexpensive way to obtain a pet with low-cost shots and neutering. Don't expect to find purebreds, and be prepared to go through applications and interviews, some of which might seem a little too personal and pushy. Don't take it personally—they have good reasons for it. Also, be sure to check the facilities and the condition of the adoptable pets. Since the animals live in close company, illness, worms, and fleas can be a problem.

Breeders. If you want a purebred cat, this is the way to go. Good breeders are extremely knowledgeable about cats in general and their breed in particular and are careful about who they sell their cats to. Beware of "bargain" purebreds and "basement breeders" (people who breed strictly for profit). A reputable breeder is interested in maintaining a high-quality animal, keeps careful records, and usually only produces one or two litters per breeding female per year.

Strays. Sometimes you don't even have to worry about finding the right cat, the right cat finds you. Many folks swear that these are the best cats to have. I'm inclined to agree, only because there's a former alley cat looking over my shoulder at this very moment. There's no adoption interviews or fees when you take in a stray, and more than likely you're saving a life. On the other hand, you'll have to cover the cost of shots, worming, neutering, and the like. Many strays have other health problems that may not show up right away and can get expensive to treat. Sometimes local humane societies will help out with initial vet care, or an area animal hospital may offer reduced rates for treating a foundling cat, but don't count on it.

Finding the Right Vet

Choosing a veterinarian for your cat is a lot like choosing a doctor for yourself. You want someone with a good bedside manner and someone you like and trust. If you have special needs, you also want a doctor who understands and keeps those needs in mind.

If you're a first-time cat owner, have recently moved to a new area, or need to find a new veterinarian, you can just try opening the Yellow Pages to "Animal Hospitals." All veterinarians go to school as many years as medical doctors and have to meet strict standards for licensing, so you're bound to find a competent and professional vet that way. But the relationship between you, your pet, and your vet is going to last for many years, and if you took the time to find just the right cat, it makes sense to find the right vet. This might be the one area where city folk have it over country folk. A small town may just have one vet, while a big city has dozens within several miles.

> The average cat lives to be about 15 years old, although some pet owners claim their cats have lived over 30 years.

Besides the Yellow Pages, here are some other sources for finding a good veterinarian:

Contact professional organizations. The American Veterinary Medical Association (AVMA) can refer you to affiliated veterinarians in your area, and the American Animal Hospital Association (AAHA) can direct you to clinics that meet its standards (see Chapter 9, "Where to Learn More"). The AVMA can also help you find feline specialists, behavior experts, veterinary eye doctors, and other professionals. Like any specialist, though, expect to pay heftier fees.

Get recommendations from other "cat people." Friends, family, and neighbors who have cats usually also have veterinarians. Take advantage of their experience, and get recommendations from them.

LOOK BEFORE YOU LEAP

Once you get a referral for a veterinarian, call up, introduce yourself, and find out when you can drop by to see the facilities and meet the doctors. Make your visit brief but thorough. Be discriminating, but don't be put off if the vet and the clinic staff can't spend a long time with you—they do have a hospital to run and patients to take care of. If you have a lot of questions and need the vet's undivided attention, the most polite thing to do is make an appointment—and offer to pay for it.

If you are going to drop by the facility and meet with the vet, here are some items to consider:

- Before you meet with the vet, determine what your needs and wants are in a vet and a veterinary hospital. Whether those needs and wants are affordable prices, the latest medical techniques and equipment, or the vet's "tableside" manner, determining your priorities ahead of time will help build a better client-veterinarian relationship.

- Ask about the practice's hours, the availability of after-hour services, and whether 24-hour-a-day emergency care is provided.

- Ask about the type of services offered, from routine physical exams to surgeries to boarding capabilities, and check the hospital's fees for each service.

- Make sure you feel comfortable with the support staff as well. A friendly, attentive staff reassures you that your pet will get the best care possible.

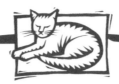

CARE AND MAINTENANCE

Imagine you had one of those really fine cars. You know—one that costs more than some folks' houses. You'd do your darnedest to keep it in top condition.

Well, a cat is a finer machine than humans can ever hope to build—and one that thinks and feels, besides. It just doesn't make sense to talk about your cat's health without the topic of proper care and maintenance coming at the top of the list.

Some folks think that because you don't have to take a cat for a walk three times a day that they're low-maintenance. But keeping your cat happy and fit does require some time and effort.

Feline Fuel:
Feeding your Cat Right

"You are what you eat" is a solid piece of common sense that city and country folk alike understand. And it's just as true for your cat as it is for you. Feed your cat a quality diet, and you're more likely to have a healthy cat.

The pet food industry is big business—and with good reason. There are well over 100 million dogs and cats living in American homes, plus who-knows-how-many more in shelters, catteries, and kennels across the country. To top it all off, you have thousands of people feeding strays. If you figure a single cat can go through some 90 pounds or more of cat food in a year, we're talking about hundreds of millions of dollars being spent annually, just to feed the kitty.

Just like human food, there are some tasty feline treats that are good for cats and some things that are basically junk food. An occasional snack of the not-so-healthy stuff shouldn't do any permanent harm but don't make it a regular part of your cat's diet.

Cats are Carnivores, but...

The wild ancestors of the modern house cat were hunters—an instinct your cat still has. Whether Tabby is bringing you gifts of demised birds and mice or pouncing on a piece of lint, she's expressing a powerful natural drive to stalk and kill prey. If you doubt that your cat is a natural-born meat eater (and predator), just take a good look at her teeth the next time she yawns. Those fangs are not designed for eating alfalfa sprouts.

The fact is your cat is so much of a carnivore, she can't survive as a vegetarian. There are certain nutrients found only in animal proteins that your cat needs. One of these nutrients is an amino acid called taurine. Without taurine, cats can go blind and develop enlarged

TALES FROM THE COUNTRY VET: FISH FETISH

The widow McCafferty's beloved cat, Patches, took ill a few years back. Patches was no spring chicken, but she wasn't exactly over-the-hill either. I'd given Patches her shots for every one of her ten years, and she'd always been a nice, plump, happy little calico. Suddenly, though, she was dropping weight.

The problem was there didn't seem to be anything wrong with her. Then I noticed a stack of canned tuna on widow McCafferty's kitchen counter. A few discreet inquiries later and I found out that Patches' diet was about half fish. A couple of phone calls to feline specialists, and my suspicions were confirmed. It's almost like cats get addicted to fish: They'll refuse to eat anything else and hold out for the good stuff, but then they may have digestive problems and weight loss if there's too much fish in their diet.

Our answer for Patches was to gradually reduce the amount of fish in her diet. In the end, Patches was limited to only two or three fish-based meals a week along with store-bought cat food for the rest of the time. There were some days she refused to eat when her beloved tuna wasn't waiting for her in her bowl in the morning; but that was usually put right by dinner-time, when she was too hungry to be picky.

hearts, which will likely give out on them well before their time. And unlike dogs, cats require a dietary source of vitamin A and a fatty acid called arachidonic acid found only in animal tissue. That's why you should never feed dog food to your cat. Dog food just doesn't have enough of the right kinds of nutrients for cats. By the pound it may be cheaper to feed dog food to your cat, but it could cost your cat her health, her sight, or even her life.

> Cats need the same basic nutrients you and I do—proteins, fats, carbohydrates, vitamins, and minerals.

Of course, that doesn't mean you should feed your cat raw meat or let her depend on hunting as her only source of food. It's been hundreds of years since cats lived in the wild, so their hunting skills are more than a little rusty. Plus, cats that hunt or eat raw or undercooked meat can pick up several kinds of diseases—including some that might get passed on to you (see the section on zoonotic diseases in Chapter 4, "What Every Cat Owner Should Know").

Home Cooking or Store-Bought Food?

The best thing about a home-cooked meal is you're the one who gets to decide what's in it. If you're a steak-and-potatoes type, then you'll broil up a nice lean Porterhouse and a batch of new reds. On the other hand, if you go for a green salad, you can pick your dinner fresh from the garden. Trying to cut down on cholesterol and salt? When you're the cook, you make the call.

Unless you are a nutritionist or dietitian, however, you should let the experts—the major pet food manufacturers—prepare the major portion of kitty's diet. Working out the right amounts and balance of foods is a difficult task. Most all food can get lumped into one or more of three categories of nutrition: protein, fat, and carbohydrate. Different kinds of animals (including people) need different proportions of protein, fat, and carbohydrate in their diets. (That's another reason why dog food isn't good for cats—dogs and cats need different percentages of fat and protein to stay healthy.) What's more, those needs change during an animal's life. A kitten has different nutritional needs than an adult cat, and they both have different needs than an old codger cat. Most pet food companies have special formulas for different levels of age and activity, and there's a whole line of prescription diets for cats with various health problems.

We've all seen a cat come running at the sound of a can opener—there's no doubt that kitty loves getting canned food. But is canned food better for cats than dry food? Not necessarily. Each type of food has its advantages and disadvantages. The most important factor is whether the food meets your cat's nutritional needs. Of course, your budget and your cat's preference also plays a role in which type of food you should choose. Store-bought cat food comes in three general forms:

- Dry cat food is also called "kibble." It's just what it sounds like: crunchy nuggets or kernels of food. Dry pet food can be stored for a long time (in a rodent-proof bin, if you have problems with mice), has no smell, and packages can be kept at room temperature for weeks without spoiling.

- Canned or "wet" cat food has a fairly long shelf life as long as it's unopened. Once you open the can, though, it doesn't hold up very well. Wet cat food usually has a pungent smell and tends to be a little bit

Care and Maintainance

What's in My Cat's Food?

Careful consumers are label readers—and that's a good place to start in figuring out just what you're feeding your cat when you buy cat food.

Many pet owners compare the nutrition information on different brands of pet food and notice that a less-expensive brand has the same nutrients as a premium cat food. What that really means is that those two foods match up in the laboratory. For example, old shoe leather might rate as high as lean chicken breasts in protein content; of course, you and your cat would both rather eat chicken. So, what you need to know is how the various nutrients match up in your cat.

You see, it's not how much of a particular nutrient there is in a can of cat food that matters but how much your cat's digestive system can take up. Cheap foods are usually made from cheap ingredients, which your cat may not digest well. Just because your cat gobbles it up and yowls for more doesn't mean a food is good for her. (Think about kids and junk food.)

The moral of the story is brand-name and specialty pet foods are made by companies that do a lot of research into pet nutrition. They're always improving their foods to keep pace with the latest information, and they use quality ingredients that have nutrients your cat can use. It may cost a little more, but it's worth it.

messy to handle. If you feed your cat wet food, any uneaten food should be picked up and discarded after 15 to 20 minutes—it's a breeding ground for bacteria that can make your cat sick. Unused portions of newly opened cans can be refrigerated in an airtight container for up to a day or two.

- Semimoist cat food also consists of individual nuggets but without the crunch of dry food. It's usually packaged in sealed canisters or individual meal-size foil pouches and is highly processed. Some semimoist cat foods are formed into interesting shapes or dyed different colors. Semimoist foods in resealable containers keep well at room temperature.

Each of these types of foods has its strong points and weak points. For instance, dry food is convenient, economical, and can be left out all day. On the other hand, the way some dry foods are formulated seems to encourage the formation of bladder stones. The rich aromas of canned food will tempt even the finickiest eater, but the crunchiness of dry food helps prevent dental plaque. Semimoist combines the convenience of dry food with the tastiness of canned food but may contain the most nonfood fillers and dyes.

> At least 26 percent of an adult cat's food (on a dry matter basis) should be protein and a minimum of nine percent should be fat.

All brand-name cat food covers the basic nutritional needs of your average cat. But if you're worried about the overall quality of the boxes, bags, and cans of feline food in the pet supplies aisle of your local market, you might want to consider one of the premium-brand foods, usually only found in pet stores or through veterinarians.

Feeding your cat store-bought food ensures that she is getting the nutrients she needs. At the same time, a home-cooked supplement to your cat's regular diet is okay if you make sure the foods you select are appropriate for cats. There's nothing wrong with getting the most out of a whole fryer by cooking up the gizzards for the cat, unless they become the major part of Tabby's diet. You see, organ meats (kidney, stomach, and even liver) are alright for your cat in moderation, but they've been linked to health problems if your cat eats too much of them. Likewise, every cat on the planet loves milk and cheese, but most cats have trouble digesting them well.

PLEASE EAT THE DAISIES

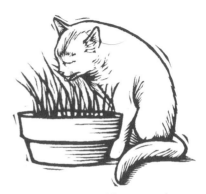

If it's green and it grows from the ground, the odds are some cat will try and eat it. This vegetarian quirk in the carnivorous cat's personality is particularly worrisome if the plants in question are your prized houseplants—or worse, if they're poisonous to your cat.

Many cat owners look at plant eating as a behavior problem—and it is if the cat is eating plants you don't want her to. Some folks assume that a cat who eats plants isn't getting enough of the right kinds of food in her diet. They're right, too—but only in the sense that what the cat needs more of in her diet is . . . plants.

The experts have a few ideas why cats eat plants. It could be to get some trace nutrients, to help with digestion, or as an emetic to help bring up swallowed hair and other nonfood items. Whatever the reason, eating vegetation is an instinctive behavior in cats; you can't stop it. So the best thing to do is point the behavior in a direction you can both live with.

Plant a "cat garden." You can find ready-made kits in pet shops and catalogs, but a more economical choice is to just do it yourself. If you're handy, you might build a fancy container out of wood or you can just use something on hand. Whatever you do, make sure you plant your cat garden in a container that doesn't tip or move easily. All you need is just a couple of inches of good potting soil and some seeds. Oat grass or catnip are good choices. You might want to keep the garden out of reach from your cats while your "crop" is coming up, but once the greens are a few inches tall, set it out and let Tabby munch at will.

Get your plants out of reach. Cats are incredibly good climbers and leapers, so putting your houseplants on stands or shelves probably won't help much. Mantels, window sills, and the like are easy landing pads for feline acrobatics. Hang plants from the ceiling, put them behind cat-proof barriers (on a sun porch closed off by glass doors, for example), or set them in locations that your cat absolutely can't jump, climb, or crawl to.

Shield your plants. If you can't get your plants out of kitty's reach, try forming a protective shield around your plants. Placing chicken wire, plant markers, or even mothballs in the soil around your plant may safeguard it from prying paws, but these barriers aren't so pretty to look at. Try adding some Spanish moss around the base of your plant to keep your cat away. Sometimes, spraying bitters on the leaves will discourage a cat from chewing. Other times, though, putting some bad-tasting substance on a plant does more harm to the plant than the cat's teeth.

Kitty Snacks and "People Food"

A well-fed cat doesn't need to snack between meals any more than you do. Too-frequent snacks will have the same effect on your cat that it can have on you: unhealthy weight gain and an imbalanced diet.

Of course, it's hard to resist the temptation to give your feline pal a treat now and then—and it's perfectly alright to give in to that temptation, assuming there's a long enough stretch of time between now and then. How long of a time depends on your cat and the kinds of treats you give her. If your cat is still eating the recommended amount of a quality cat food every day and isn't overweight, then you're probably not giving her too many treats. If, on the other hand, your cat is chowing down on tasty but not-so-nutritious snacks and is either getting plumper or turning her nose up at dinner, it's time to change your strategy.

Store-bought cat treats tend not to be packed with good nutrition. Their main purpose is the same as human treats: to taste good—real good—and that's about it. "Gourmet" cat snacks usually have less artificial colors and fillers in them but still aren't meant to be fed as a regular part of Tabby's diet. The good thing about "gourmet" treats is the cost: They're usually so expensive that cat owners won't overfeed them to their cats!

A question vets hear all the time is, "Can I feed my cat people food?" There's very little that people eat that cats shouldn't (or won't), so that's not really so much of a problem. (Cat owners should be careful about feeding dairy products their pets. Although cats love dairy products, many don't digest them well and may get sick.) The question once again is nutritional balance. Just like with home cooking, feeding your cat leftovers or using people food for snacks may not be providing her with the right nutrients in the right amounts.

Still, people food might provide some of the healthiest snacks for cats. If you give your cat some scrambled egg or a couple of pieces of pasta, at least you know what's in it. And you might be surprised what your cat will eat. Cat owners report their pets begging for predictable tidbits such as fish and chicken as well as unexpected ones, including tomatoes and cantaloupe.

WATER, WATER EVERYWHERE

Your cat needs about an ounce of water per pound of body weight every day. That doesn't sound like much, but it adds up: An average-size cat would need more than a gallon of water every week.

Of course, cats get water by drinking. But there's another important source of water for your cat: the food she eats. The more water there is in her food, the less she needs to drink. Canned cat food is more expensive because you're buying water along with the food (up to 75 percent of wet cat food is water) and paying a little more for the container. Dry cat food has much less water (perhaps 10 percent by weight), which means a cat whose diet consists of only dry food has to drink a lot more.

Dehydration (not enough water in the body) is a serious problem for any living creature, and cats are especially prone to it. A cat can go without food for days, losing up to 40 percent of her body weight, and still survive. But a loss of body water of only 10 to 15 percent can kill her. Other liquids—like milk, if it doesn't make your cat sick—are a good source of water, but nothing beats the real thing. Be sure your cat always has plenty of clean, fresh water available at all times.

LOOK SHARP, BE SHARP: GROOMING YOUR CAT

Ever wonder why some cats always look sleek and beautiful and others look like ... well, like something the cat dragged in? While it's true that some cats (like some people) are just born with "good hair," a lot of it has to do with grooming.

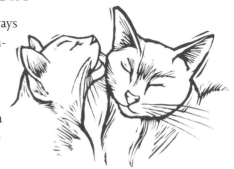

Care and Maintainance

Now, cats are fastidious critters. They tend to take care of themselves pretty well, always licking their fur to keep it clean and in its proper place. But any cat can go from Fluffy to Scruffy without a little help from her human pals.

LONGHAIR VS. SHORTHAIR CATS

The magnificent coat of a champion Persian is truly a work of art. But you'd better believe that it took hours of regular grooming to get it—and keep it—that way. It's common sense that the more hair there is to take care of, the more work that goes into it. The fluffier the cat's hair, the more likely it is to form mats, too.

> Kittens began grooming each other and their mothers when they are only three weeks of age, and this behavior continues into adulthood between friendly cats.

These thick tangles of hair can be painful and even tear a cat's skin if the mats get bad enough. Mats get embarrassing for a cat, too, since the only way to get rid of really bad ones is to shave them off. Nothing looks more uncomfortable than a cat who has been shaved.

It's not that shorthair cats don't need regular grooming or never get mats—they do. It's just that their shorter, coarser outer coat requires lower maintenance than a long, silky coat. A shorthair cat who's diligent about her own grooming routine can do a lot to make up for an owner who's a little lazy with the brush and comb. But regular grooming is still a must for both longhair and shorthair cats.

Cats use their tongue and teeth for grooming. Every time Tabby goes into her contortionist bathing routine, she's swallowing hair. The more hair she has (and the more grooming she does), the more hair she swallows. Hair doesn't digest and can clump up in a cat's stomach and intestines to form hairballs. The least dangerous, but still rather

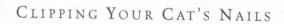

CLIPPING YOUR CAT'S NAILS

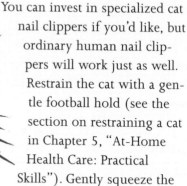

You can invest in specialized cat nail clippers if you'd like, but ordinary human nail clippers will work just as well. Restrain the cat with a gentle football hold (see the section on restraining a cat in Chapter 5, "At-Home Health Care: Practical Skills"). Gently squeeze the cat's toe between your thumb and forefinger, extending the nail. Gently clip off the sharp tip, being careful to stay in the clear portion toward the end of the nail (you should be able to see the reddish "quick" through the nail; don't cut this far or you'll cause discomfort and bleeding). Repeat with each toe.

No cat enjoys having her nails trimmed, but if you start them as kittens it will be easier when they're adults. Also be sure to play with your cat's feet and toes for fun sometimes, too; otherwise she'll always know you're going to cut her nails the minute you take hold of her foot.

unpleasant, side effect of hairballs is your cat coughing them up—quite often at times or in places you'd much rather she didn't. On a more serious note, a lot of swallowed hair can actually block your cat's intestines, calling for an operation to save her life. The bottom line, as they say in the city, is to invest a few dollars in a brush and comb—and use them.

Do I Need a Professional Groomer?

Because longhair cats need regular grooming (with daily grooming really being the best), you might want to consult your budget before answering this question. But even if you have the means to bring your longhair cat to a professional groomer weekly, you should still have grooming tools on hand at home—and know how to use them. You never know when your cat might get into something that needs to be combed out right away or when she might need a touch-up between trips to the groomer.

The main advantages of a professional groomer are training, skill, and experience. A good groomer can get your cat's coat looking spiffy quickly and humanely, with a minimum amount of trauma. Really bad mats and tangles can be dealt with at home, but if you've never done that sort of thing before, you run the risk of injuring your cat—an injury that will probably need veterinary attention. Such grooming problems are probably best left to the professionals, too.

Even folks who learn to wield a slicker brush and metal comb with a good amount of expertise will turn to a professional groomer from time to time. It could be for a bad mat or tangle, during a particularly heavy period of shedding, or just to get the full treatment so that Tabby looks her best.

Tools and Tips for At-Home Grooming

Every cat owner needs some groom-ing supplies. A metal comb is the most essential basic grooming tool. Sturdy stainless steel combs with wide-set, round teeth are widely available and reasonably priced. A slicker brush has bristles that look like dozens of tiny bent nails. They

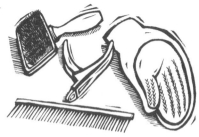

resemble the rasps on a cat's tongue and serve the same purpose in grooming. Most cats enjoy the sensation of the slicker brush and the metal comb—unless, of course, you hit a tangle or mat.

You may also want to invest in a flea comb, particularly if you let your cat outdoors, live in a year-round flea climate (like southern Florida or Louisiana), or have other pets who go outdoors. Flea combs look like metal combs but with very fine teeth set close together. Flea combs can be used for regular grooming, as a "touch-up" after the slicker brush or metal comb. Grooming mitts fit over your whole hand and let you work a larger surface while petting your cat.

Here are a few tips for home grooming:

Make it fun. Most cats love being stroked and enjoy the feeling of light grooming. It's good social behavior—cats who get along well will blissfully groom each other for long periods of time. When it's time to do some grooming, approach your cat in a friendly way, and intersperse the grooming strokes with some regular petting.

Use restraint. It's okay to restrain your cat (gently!) as long as she doesn't start to panic, but be sure to restrain yourself, too. Don't try to force your cat to sit still or stay in an awkward or uncomfortable position for too long. And be careful not to get too exuberant in your grooming strokes. Think about how much you don't like having your hair pulled, then imagine what it's like to have hair getting pulled all over your body.

Know when to quit. You may not be able to groom your cat completely in one session. That's okay. If you get her back and tail, and then she starts to fight you, give up and try finishing up in a day or two. It's better to have a half-dozen five-minute grooming sessions spread out over a week and a happy cat than one 25-minute battle and a cat who runs and hides at the sight of the brush.

Care and Maintainance

Get professional help. If your cat has a bad mat or tangle—or gets something nasty on her fur—put in a call to your veterinarian or professional groomer. If your cat just doesn't seem to be cooperating with home grooming, schedule an appointment with a professional. While you're there, ask for some tips and a demonstration of basic techniques. Groomers are usually happy to do this for clients; there's nothing more annoying for a groomer than having to constantly shave out and untangle bad mats. The cat suffers, and the groomer is more likely to get bitten or scratched.

BATHS AND HAIRCUTS

Except for removing a mat or performing a medical procedure, there is almost no other reason to shave a cat's hair. Cats are built to have a full coat of hair—taking it away can throw off regulation of their body temperature and exposes the usually protected skin underneath.

Trimming a longhair cat's coat for appearances and to prevent tangles is fine, but it should be done by a professional groomer.

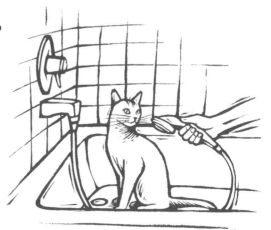

It's usually not necessary to bathe a cat, either, since they do so well keeping themselves clean. Sometimes, though, a bath is called for to treat or control fleas, to clean up an adventurous feline explorer, to treat a skin condition, or to remove a noxious or dangerous mess from your cat's fur. The squeamish, the inexperienced, and the uncertain should probably let a veterinarian or groomer take care of these mandatory baths. For those who want to try it at home, here are several bath basics.

Be prepared. Lay out your bathing supplies ahead of time. You'll need a good pet shampoo (get medicated shampoos for fleas or skin conditions from your vet, not over-the-counter); a large, fluffy towel; a brush and comb; and either a hand-held shower head or plastic tumbler for wetting and rinsing. It's a good idea to comb out your cat's hair before bathing, if possible, especially for longhairs. If you know how, now is the time to trim your cat's nails. (Note: You can protect your cat's eyes during a bath with a neutral ophthalmic ointment available from your veterinarian.)

Ready your bathing stations. Use a large sink with a dish sprayer attachment or the bathtub. Start the water before you put the cat in, and make sure it's not too hot or too cold. A comfortable temperature for your hands should work fine. You're going to get wet, splattered with suds, and possibly jumped on by an upset, sopping cat, so dress appropriately in clothes that can get soiled yet protect you from scratches.

Before you add the cat. Bathing a cat is often a two-person job—one to restrain and one to bathe—but you can do it yourself. Either way, practice restraint techniques on dry land before the bath. With one hand, grasp your cat firmly but gently at the base of the neck or on the scruff, pressing down slightly. See how well you can reach the various parts of your cat's body with the other hand. Figure out when and how you'll have to change grips during the bath. Get your bathing routine down step-by-step before the cat is in the tub or sink; otherwise, Tabby will be able to make a break for it in your moment of hesitation or confusion.

Start the suds. Wet your cat down, starting from the head and working your way to the tail. Apply the shampoo the same way, lather, and rinse thoroughly. (Read the label directions on medicated shampoos carefully. Some require 5 to 15 minutes before rinsing in order to be effective.) Thorough rinsing is important. Leftover soap residue can

Care and Maintainance

irritate your cat's skin or be swallowed when your cat licks her fur. Rinsing also gets rid of fleas and other parasites that are immobilized—but not killed—by the bath.

Dry and fluff. Gently squeeze excess water out of your cat's fur, wrap her up in a large fluffy towel, and dry her off. If she'll stand for it, you can comb out any tangles right away; otherwise, wait until she's dried off and settled down. If you're lucky, your cat may tolerate the sound and feel of a blow-dryer. Don't count on it, though—many cats are terrified by them. This is not something to discover right after a bath. See how your cat reacts to the blow-dryer on a nonbath day. If she's scared witless, stick with a towel. You might be able to gradually get her used to the sound and feel (especially if you begin regular baths in kittenhood)—and then again, you might not!

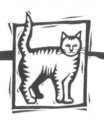

An Ounce of Prevention

Sometimes it seems like we have things backwards, like paying doctors when we get sick. In China, the traditional country doctors get paid for keeping folks well—now that makes more sense.

The truth is everyone is bound to get a little under the weather some time. But good doctors—and good vets—know there are tried-and-true ways to keep from getting sick. Some of them are just plain common sense, and some of them take a little thought and planning—like getting shots or accident-proofing your home—but all of them are certainly worth that proverbial "pound of cure."

Cat-Proofing:
Making Your Home Safe

We all know to keep dangerous substances away from children, and it's important to remember that we should be even more careful with cats. We all know the old saying about what curiosity did to the cat. Because they are smaller, more mobile, and have more sensitive noses than children, cats are more likely to investigate, getting into things that can be dangerous. To prevent your cat's curiosity from becoming fatal, there are a few household dangers to look out for.

Drapery, blind, and electrical cords. To your cat's eye, the dangling end of a drapery or blind cord is an open invitation to play—and possibly to disaster. Even just crawling between drapes or blinds and the window (an all-time favorite feline pastime) can land Tabby in a tangle. Cats who get caught in the loops of pull-cords panic. At the very least, the blinds or drapery rod will come down with a crash. At worst, a cat can strangle, do fatal internal damage, or actually get so worked up that his heart gives out. For maximum safety, tie or wrap all window cords well out of feline reach.

Electrical and telephone cords pose something of a tangling threat but more often are dangerous on account of chewing. It might be the taste or texture of the plastic coating, but for some reason, a lot of cats can't resist nibbling. There's not much direct danger in chewing phone cords (except when you try to make a call on a line that's been put out of commission by your cat) since there's very little current run-ning through them.

Electrical cords are another story altogether, of course. Wherever possible, run the cords under rugs and carpets or behind furniture that sits flush to the floor and wall. If a cord has to be run where a cat can reach it, buy some inexpensive plastic conduit, which is available at most hardware and building supply stores. For a larger investment, you can get flat strips of heavy-duty vinyl that not only protect the electrical cords, but also keep the cords flush to the floor to prevent tripping.

Occasionally, a very determined cat will make his way through all the physical barriers. Treating the cords with a bad-tasting substance like bitter apple might do the trick. A little behavior modification, using positive reinforcement (see Chapter 7, "Behavior and Training"), will help, too.

Cleaning fluids, antifreeze, and other poisons. We don't just buy cleaners to get our house clean; we want it disinfected and smelling nice, too. Unfortunately, some of the very products we buy to sanitize and deodorize pet areas are outright dangerous for your cat.

Pine-based cleaners and those containing phenol (the most popular being Lysol disinfectant) are particularly toxic to cats and shouldn't be used on food bowls or in pet areas, sleeping quarters, or litter boxes. Of course, any cleaning compound can be poisonous if taken internally, so keep everything secured in a locking cabinet. (A simple spring latch won't keep a determinedly curious cat out.)

Ethylene glycol is the stuff that makes antifreeze work. It just so happens that it also smells and tastes very sweet. A significant number of cats and dogs—and even small children—suffer from ethylene glycol poisoning every winter. Because it's present in large amounts in almost every home and is very often fatal if swallowed, antifreeze and other products containing ethylene glycol should be considered dangerous and never left where pets or children can get to them.

Cats who go outdoors run the added risk of lapping up antifreeze spills and drips, an especially tempting thing for a thirsty cat to do since those puddles of tasty liquid don't freeze on cold days. You can protect your own cat (and other outdoor cats and strays) by immediately cleaning up and washing down any of your own spills or drips, or you can purchase one of the new nontoxic brands of antifreeze that contain propylene glycol rather than ethylene glycol. It's important to also keep in mind that once your cat leaves your property, there's no guarantee that everyone else in the area is going to be equally careful.

In general, anything that's toxic to you will be poisonous to your cat as well. The rule of thumb is: If you'd keep it out of reach of a child, keep it out of reach of your cat.

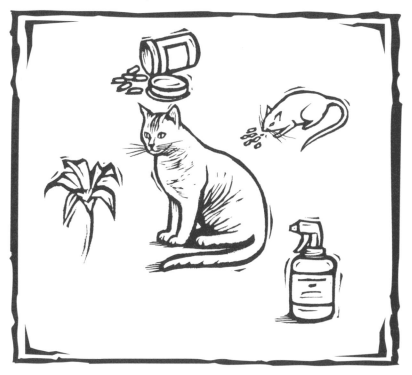

The Animal
Poison Control Hotline

"My cat is a chowhound—she never misses a meal," one cat owner recalls. "So when she didn't come running at dinnertime, I knew something was very wrong. I found her under the bed, and when I coaxed her out, she was staggering and drooling. I was terrified. She had this funny smell, which I recognized as the cleaning fluid I kept in my linen closet. I ran to the closet, and I found the door open and the can of cleaning fluid spilled on the floor.

"The problem is, we live a good 30 minutes from the nearest veterinarian. I didn't know how long she had been poisoned, and I wasn't sure that she had another half hour to spare. Then I remembered about the hotline—and it saved my cat's life."

The ASPCA National Animal Poison Control Center (also called the Animal Poison Hotline) is operated by the University of Illinois College of Veterinary Medicine (2001 South Lincoln Avenue, Urbana, Illinois 61801). There is a charge for calls, and you have two options for payment and fees:

- Call 1 (800) 548-2423. There's a $30 flat fee, chargeable to a credit card (have your charge card ready).

- Call 1 (900) 680-0000. The charge is $20 for the first five minutes, $2.95 per minute thereafter; charges will appear on your next phone bill.

An Ounce of Prevention

Poisonous plants. A cat chewing on your houseplants is more than an annoyance, it can be dangerous or even fatal to the cat.

Technically, any plant that makes your cat sick when eaten is a "poisonous" plant. (Nearly all cats will eat grass or plants to purge themselves, however, so vomiting alone may not be a reliable sign of poisoning.) Still, some plants have particularly serious effects. The list of potentially poisonous plants includes: apricot (pits), azalea, buttercup, caladium, calla lily, castorbean, cherry (twigs, leaves, bark, fruit, and stones), chrysanthemums, crocus, daffodil (bulbs), daphne (berries), holly, hydrangea, iris (leaves, roots, and fleshy parts), ivy, lily-of-the-valley (leaves, flowers, roots), mistletoe (especially the berries), mushrooms, narcissus (bulbs), oak (acorns, young shoots, and leaves), oleander, peach (pits), philodendron, poison ivy, potatoes ("eyes" and sprouts from the eyes; the edible part of the potato is safe), privet, rhubarb (leaves), rosary pea (shiny red and black seeds), star of Bethlehem (bulb), string-of-pearls, sumac, and sweet pea (seeds and pods).

Dieffenbachia is a fairly common houseplant that also goes by the name of "dumb cane." The dumb cane is aptly named. Chewing dieffenbachia can actually paralyze your cat's mouth, making it impossible for him to eat and drink. The name "dumb cane" comes from the most noticeable effect of this paralysis on people: They can't talk.

Poinsettias (Christmas flowers) belong to the nightshade family—flowers notorious in fact and literature for their deadly properties. A study a few years back seemed to show that poinsettias—long believed to be dangerously toxic to cats and dogs—don't make cats any sicker than many plants considered nonpoisonous. Still, it's always safest to keep cats away from any houseplant, just to be sure.

Windows, balconies, and screens. "High-rise syndrome" might sound like some sort of pop psychology explanation for violent crime, but it actually describes an epidemic that hits a number of cats every year, especially in warmer weather. "High-rise syndrome" is a collection of various injuries that are the result of a fall from a high window.

Amazingly, there are many stories of cats surviving falls from several flights up. But there are far more who fell and didn't make it. The saddest part of it is nearly all of those falls could have been prevented.

Every window that you plan to open needs to have a screen. And not just any screen. A cat-proof screen has to fit the window frame securely enough to stay firmly in place when confronted by ten or more pounds of cat. When ordering or replacing screens, use a heavy-duty grade of hardware cloth since ordinary screens can be easily torn by claws or teeth. Even a fall from a second- or third-story window can cause serious injury or death, so inspect all screens regularly, especially toward the end of winter in cold-weather areas of the country. Screens can warp, tear, or fatigue in the off-season.

Some city cat owners think letting Tabby out on the balcony of their apartment is a safe way to give him some fresh air and sunshine. Actually, a good number of "high-rise syndrome" cats were stalking moths, birds, or other irresistible things on an upper-floor balcony, when an ill-timed pounce or missed step sent them over the railing. Even a leash or tether on an open balcony doesn't ensure your cat's safety. A panicked cat dangling from by his collar or harness can be strangled, seriously injured, or squirm loose and fall anyway.

Good Toy, Bad Toy: Playtime Safety

It's like something right out of a Norman Rockwell painting: a fuzzy little kitten tumbling around with a ball of yarn. Well, old Norman apparently never had to rush his cat to the vet for emergency surgery to get a couple of feet of that yarn unraveled from the poor cat's digestive tract. Yarn and string can turn even the most disinterested cats wide-eyed and playful but should never be left where cats or kittens can get at it on their own. Besides choking and intestinal blockage dangers, a cat who gets tangled up in string or yarn—even during supervised play—can panic and injure himself, possibly fatally. Take special care to keep sewing thread and dental floss out of feline reach; it's much finer and can become imbedded in the tissues of your cat's mouth, stomach, and intestines.

Cats will turn anything shiny, crinkly, or small enough to bat across the floor into a toy. Since Tabby doesn't have hands, he has to pick up these makeshift toys in his mouth, where they can be easily swallowed (or if not easily swallowed, can cause choking). At best, a foreign object in your cat's digestive system can trigger vomiting or diarrhea, but it can often be much worse. Keep things like paper clips, foil, and rubber bands safely tucked away.

Cellophane candy wrappers are particularly dangerous. Cats can't resist the crinkly texture, and the sugary residue makes them a cinch to get eaten. The wrappers can liquefy in your cat's stomach, coating the lining and blocking the uptake of nutrients from food.

What makes for a good cat toy? Here's what to look for:

Something sturdy. If it can get tossed, thrown, gnawed, clawed, batted, kicked, licked, and repeatedly pounced on without coming apart, it's a good cat toy. Catnip-filled toys encourage play, but most cats like to eat catnip and will try to lick and chew their way to that scrumptious herbal filling. Catnip toys made from light fabric or felt will most likely be in shreds—and the shreds in your cat's tummy—within a week. Ditto for plastic or vinyl toys that can be chewed up, cracked, or shattered.

No (re)movable parts. Catnip mousies with yarn tails; crinkly caterpillars with bug eyes; oversized plush "bumblebees" with glued-on felt features, and plastic mesh balls with tantalizing little bells inside are four of the more popular cat toys. But they share a common failing: small and potentially dangerous parts that come off. If you can pull or peel a part or decoration off of a cat toy, the odds are your cat can, too. In fact, go ahead and try it with all your cat's toys—it's better to have some catnip mice without tails than make a trip to the vet to get the tails out of your cat's stomach.

> Kittens aren't usually susceptible to the effects of catnip until they're about three months old. Then about 50 percent of cats actually react to the plant.

Something fun. A toy just isn't a toy if your cat won't play with it. Cat owners are often disappointed—and frequently annoyed—to find that the $100 worth of custom cat toys they bring home get passed over for a piece of crumpled paper or a simple Ping Pong ball. Cats like games that involve what they do best: climbing, running, leaping, stalking, and pouncing. Pick toys that encourage those behaviors, and your cat is bound to use them. That's the allure of the Ping Pong ball—it rolls and hops and skitters away when your cat pounces on it, encouraging batting and chasing. Cats see moving edges better than stationary objects, so toys that wiggle, bob, or weave fascinate them and trigger the stalking and hunting reflexes.

An Ounce of Prevention

SHOULD I HAVE AN INDOOR CAT?

Perhaps nothing is as pitiful as the wail of a cat who wants to be on the other side of a door. When it's the front door, many of us take that to mean that our cats won't be truly happy unless they go out-doors. But, then again, most cats make the same kind of racket when they want to come inside (or, for that matter, when they want to get through any door). Do cats really want to go outside? Do they need to? And even if the answer to both questions is "yes," is it really in their best interest?

Safe at home vs. the great outdoors. "It's more natural for my cat to be outside," argue many cat owners. "Dogs go out every day—why not cats?"

Let's talk about the second point first. The main reason dogs are walked is elimination, followed closely by exercise. Only the smallest dogs can get enough running indoors. Dogs are pack hunters, which means they work cooperatively to run their quarry to exhaustion. That can take all day, which means dogs have a natural instinct to run ... and run ... and run. You need a lot of open space for that kind of work. Cats, on the other hand, are "ambush hunters." They rely on relatively short bursts of very fast running. A hallway of any decent length provides plenty of room for that. That combined with the instinct to bury wastes (which is why cats will use a litter box) adds up to no pressing reason to take a cat outdoors.

Of course, fresh air and sunshine are good for anyone—human or cat. But is the outdoor life really more "natural" for your cat? Sure, his wild ancestors lived outdoors. But that was a few thousand years and several hundred generations ago. To top it all off, those ancestors lived in the arid regions of the Mideast—a far cry from the climate and surroundings of the United States today. Once cats were domesti-cated, they stopped being completely "natural"; once they were

Cats and the Law: Is Your Cat a Stray?

Most of us think of "leash laws" in terms of dogs. But many cities, towns, and even counties have revamped these animal control laws to include all kinds of pets. Some cat owners have resisted leash and licensing laws for cats, but the trend seems to be headed that way.

You may be surprised to find out that anytime your cat leaves your property by himself, he's technically considered a stray. That means local animal control authorities can pick him up, hold him for the required time (which can range from as long as a week or two to as short as 24 hours), then dispose of him however the law allows (this includes euthanasia).

Check with your town, county, and state animal control agencies to see what the laws are in your area. The odds are, a free-roaming feline is breaking the law.

uprooted from their original habitat, they had to do their best to adapt instincts honed over tens of thousands of years of living in Middle Eastern deserts to their new circumstances. Some of those circumstances—the bitter cold of a Midwestern winter, dogs and wild animals that will turn them from hunter to hunted, and speeding cars and trucks, just to name a few—they can never really adapt to.

The not-so-great outdoors. What's waiting for your cat, just outside your front door? Yes, there are trees and grass and all the sights, sounds, smells, and joys of nature—good things for all of us to savor. But there are also vicious animals, cruel people, traffic, disease, and animal control officers (who may be within their legal right to grab and impound your cat, if he steps off your property). The only reliable way to keep your cat safe from all of these deadly hazards is to keep him indoors.

Truth be told, country cats aren't necessarily safer outdoors than city cats. Sure, there's a lot more chance of being hit by a car or mauled by a stray dog in the city. But out in the country, we've got some predators that run bigger, quicker, and savvier than a feral city dog. We've also got less light on the roads, making strays harder to see—and easier to hit—and usually more kinds of disease-bearing insects, such as ticks.

A whole host of serious and fatal feline diseases need contact with infected cats—or areas where infected cats hang out a lot—to spread. Feline immunodeficiency virus (FIV), which causes a breakdown in the cat's disease-fighting immune system, is mostly passed by bites from infected cats. And feline leukemia virus (FeLV) generally requires prolonged close contact with an infected cat, such as sharing litter boxes or food and water bowls, or mutual grooming. Time and again, the risks for disease are minor or negligible for indoor cats, significantly higher for outdoor or indoor/outdoor cats. Cat owners— especially those with young children—should be particularly aware that outdoor cats are more likely to pick up diseases and parasites that can effect humans, from minor annoyances like fleas to more serious illness like Lyme tick disease to extremely dangerous conditions like rabies.

Going outside safely. Just because it's safest for your cat to live indoors and not roam free doesn't mean he can never see the light of day except through the window. A leash and harness (not a collar) is a fairly safe way for both you and your cat to get some fresh air and sunshine. Walking on a leash is an acquired taste that some cats will never acquire, though. Regular experience from kittenhood helps, and some leash-trained cats will even request a walk. Of course, a cat on a leash is still at risk for picking up fleas—and for encounters with unleashed cats and dogs in the neighborhood.

Building a cat run is actually not as hard as it sounds. Runs must be enclosed on all sides (including the top) and solidly anchored and constructed. Screens should be the heaviest grade of outdoor mesh, and walls should extend a few inches below the ground to prevent cats from digging their way out—or other animals from digging their way in. If the run isn't built attached to your home, with a pet door or other door leading indoors, be sure it includes some sort of heated, waterproof shelter for your cat to retreat to in case of inclement weather.

It's especially important for a run or other outdoor enclosure to have a roof. Cats are terrific climbers and leapers, and even an eight- to ten-foot wall may not hold them, especially if there are screens to hook onto. The roof and walls of the run provide another kind of security, too—they keep other things out. Openings in roof or walls let unfriendly or dangerous animals, people, and things into an area that your cat may not be able to escape.

Free-roaming cats get into loud, late night spats with other cats, chew or dig up neighbors' plants, kill local birds (but also may help control the local rodent population), and bury their wastes in other people's gardens. While some folks—and some cat owners—see these as minor annoyances, many other folks see them as much more serious problems. If your cat gets into a fight, it may do more than wake the neighbors because of the yowling and screaming. The superficial scratches you may see on his face or back aren't so bad. But he may also have bite wounds that close up quickly, sealing in dirt and germs and creating a painful abscess several days later. Bites during fights also seem to be the main way to spread feline immunodeficiency virus. Unaltered cats that roam free also contribute to pet overpopulation, a problem that fills animal shelters to capacity and beyond, resulting in millions of dogs and cats being "put to sleep" every year.

Fix It:
The Case for Neutering and Spaying

Neutering and spaying (otherwise known as "altering" or "fixing" your cat) are routine operations that a skilled vet can usually do in 30 minutes or less. Both neutering a male cat (also called orchidectomy or castration) and spaying a female cat (also known as complete hysterectomy or ovariohysterectomy) make the cats sterile (incapable of producing offspring). Neutering and spaying are usually done around the ages of five to seven months, when pet cats are raised from kittens. Adults can be altered at any age, unless they're too weak or ill or have some health problem that makes surgery too risky.

> One breeding pair of cats can produce over 100,000 descendants in 10 years.

In recent years, so-called "early" neutering and spaying has become popular, especially among animal shelters. Kittens as young as seven weeks undergo surgical sterilization. In the past, the prevailing wisdom said that anesthesia and surgery on kittens that young was dangerous and probably foolhardy. Further, neutering and spaying that young would be expected to have serious long-range effects on the cat's health. As it turns out, that doesn't seem to be the case. Seven-week-old kittens are up and playing within a few hours after surgery and don't seem to have any significantly different side effects than cats neutered or spayed at seven months old—the more typical age for altering.

Neutering and spaying do four good things for your cat:

- Your cat will live longer. On average, cats who are neutered and spayed have double the life expectancy of unaltered cats.

- Your cat will be happier. You only have to see (and hear) a cat in heat once to know that she isn't having a good time. Male cats who haven't been neutered can detect a female cat in heat from great distances and will escape and roam (and get into fights) to find her. Neutered and spayed cats are much more content.

- Your cat will be healthier. Believe it or not, intact cats (cats that haven't been neutered or spayed) run a higher risk of certain diseases, including some kinds of cancer. This is especially true for female cats. Pyometra is an infection of the cat's uterus that can be fatal if not caught and treated in time. Since the treatment includes spaying the cat anyway, that should be reason enough to spay your female cat while she's still healthy. If that doesn't convince you, try this: Having even one heat cycle dramatically increases a female cat's risk of mammary tumors, which is the feline equivalent of breast cancer. The longer your cat goes without being spayed, the greater the danger.

- You'll prevent homelessness and save lives. We really don't know how many stray and homeless cats there are in the United States, but estimates range from a few million to tens of millions. What we do know is that several million cats are put to sleep in animal shelters every year because there aren't enough homes for them all.

VISIT THE VET

Cats live an average of 12 to 15 years, but more and more are living into their late teens and even early 20s. Those kind of rich, full lives don't usually happen without regular visits to the veterinarian.

Being a pet owner has some extra challenges when it comes to keeping your pet healthy. Most important, your cat can't talk. He can't tell you when he's feeling a little funny, having tightness in his chest, getting twinges in the litter box, or experiencing blurred vision. Since those are all important early warnings of more serious problems, it would be good if there was some way to detect them.

While a vet can't get your cat to talk, he or she can pick up many of those early warnings in other ways—early warnings that can catch problems before they turn serious. But that can only happen if your bring your cat in for regular checkups.

As cats age, there will likely be more for the vet to do at checkup time. For example, there will be blood samples taken (and possibly urine or stool samples, too) to check on the health of internal organs. Your vet can also keep you up-to-date on an aging cat's changing nutritional needs and stay on top of dental plaque, tooth loss, and gum disease.

Vaccinations

Kittens get a series of shots. Adults get annual boosters. But what exactly are vaccinations, and how do they help keep cats healthy? Here's how most vaccines work. Researchers find the germ causing the disease—for example, the virus that causes feline distemper. Next they produce a harmless, noncontagious version of the virus. This form of the virus is used to vaccinate healthy cats. The vaccine triggers the cat's disease-fighting immune system, which attacks and destroys the virus. This exposure "primes" the immune system so that if the same virus shows up again—even the dangerous, contagious version—it will be destroyed before it can cause illness.

Vaccines protect your cat from common diseases, mostly caused by viruses. When a virus invades an animal's body, no medicine can kill it. You can give a cat with a virus things like antibiotics from now until doomsday, and it won't cure the disease (although the antibiotics will help treat or control infections that might start as a result of the cat's being sick with the virus). Viral diseases just have to run their course, after which the victim is often immune for life. Vaccines (usually with regular booster shots) provide your cat with the benefits of being immune without actually having to suffer through the disease.

Vaccines can't cure diseases caused by viruses. Going back to feline distemper for a moment, if a cat has already contracted this disease, the vaccine won't stop it. Vaccines also can't prevent every viral disease every time. No vaccine is 100 percent effective, so every once in awhile a cat who has all his shots will still get sick with something he's supposed to be protected against. Some diseases, like FIV, are caused by viruses that shut down the immune system when they first enter the cat's body. In those cases, the vaccine can't do its job because its tools (the disease-fighting system of the cat's body) have been taken away.

Get your cat's shots from a veterinarian or animal hospital. At the bare minimum, cats should be up-to-date on their rabies shot and distemper-combination vaccine. The combination shot usually carries protection against feline distemper (panleukopenia) and common upper respiratory diseases that cause cold- or flu-like symptoms in your cat (feline viral rhinotracheitis and calicivirus). Any cat being vaccinated for the first time usually needs a series of shots, spaced a couple of weeks apart. Young kittens don't have full-blown immune systems and need boosters every few weeks until they're three or four months old, and then annually after that. (The exception is rabies vaccinations; a kitten usually receives one shot given at three to four months of age. Rabies boosters are given annually or every three years, depending on the type of vaccine or the requirements of state law.) Most vaccines are given under the cat's skin and don't hurt much at all.

Vaccines for other cat diseases have been around since the mid-1980s, particularly the one for feline leukemia virus (FeLV). FeLV (or FeLeuk, as it's sometimes known) attacks a cat's white blood cells and can produce a kind of cancer. Research shows that most cats exposed to FeLV don't get sick, but even infected cats who appear healthy can still pass the virus on to other cats. Once a cat does get sick from FeLV, though, the odds are almost 100 percent that it will be a fatal illness.

The FeLV is a funny creature—it doesn't last long outside of a cat's body, unless it stays a little moist. So the most common way FeLV gets passed is prolonged close contact between a healthy cat and infected cat—things like mutual grooming, or sharing food, water, and litter boxes. This also means that the FeLV vaccine may not be necessary for a cat that is never exposed to FeLV-infected cats. A simple blood test can determine if your cat (or any new cat you're thinking of taking into your home) is infected. If not, keeping your FeLV-free cats indoors and away from FeLV-infected cats is probably all the protection they need (outdoor or indoor/outdoor cats are a different story). If your cat tests positive for FeLV, the vaccine won't help, either; vaccines don't kill the virus, they only protect uninfected cats from getting it.

Feline infectious peritonitis (FIP) is also a fatal cat disease caused by a virus. There are blood tests for FIP, but they're not as conclusive as the FeLV tests. There is an FIP vaccine, but the jury is still out on how safe and effective it is. Your veterinarian can help you figure out if your cat is at risk for FIP and if the potential benefits of the FIP vaccine outweigh the added risks.

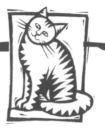

WHAT EVERY CAT OWNER
SHOULD KNOW

"Forewarned is forearmed," goes a fine old folk saying. In a little less flowery terms that simply means if you know what to expect—or what to look for—you're going to be better prepared to handle whatever comes your way.

We can tell if a person is feeling poorly by his facial expression . . . or because he's one of those folks who loves to tell you about every little ache and pain. Well, a cat's skin is completely covered in fur, she only has a few facial expressions, and she can't talk, so it's up to you to know the subtle—and not-so-subtle—signs that something could be wrong.

Whenever something isn't quite right with your cat, there are usually early warning signs. Unfortunately, the signs may be so slight when they first show up, you can easily miss them. Other times, you might notice something a little different about your cat, but it appears harmless—and even cute. Keep in mind, the early warning signs may build up so slowly over such a long time that by the time you notice them they aren't early warnings anymore.

When your cat has a serious illness, nothing is worse than 20/20 hindsight—that terrible feeling of not seeing something coming when all the signals were there. To help spare you from all of that, here are some important things to look out for.

Changes in behavior. Has your usually friendly cat become more moody, shy, or touchy about being petted lately? Or has your usually moody or shy cat become noticeably more friendly? Any kind of personality change in a cat could be a signal of a developing health problem. New behaviors or increased frequency of behaviors may also be an early warning, such as a cat that never drank from the faucet suddenly learning the trick or an "itchy" cat scratching or rubbing her ears more often. Likewise, if your cat seems thirstier (drinks more often or for longer periods of time), she could be telling you she's got a kidney problem, early diabetes, or simply that it's a little too dry in the house.

You see, it's important to stress here that these behavioral early warnings are just that: warnings. They don't necessarily mean there's a

Tales from the Country Vet: Pansy Gets Happy

In a quaint little animal shelter lived a portly tortie named Pansy. The old girl had four big rooms on the second floor of an old Victorian house to roam, complete with climbers, hidey-holes, perches, and banks of sunny windows. There were also plenty of other cats and humans around for her to play with, but she would have none of them. Pansy was a loner.

That is, she was a loner. I was strolling through the shelter one afternoon, when I heard a loud but unfamiliar chirrup. I glanced around to see if any of the usual suspects were looking for a favor. No dice. Then I heard the chirruping again and saw a pair of emerald eyes peering out from Pansy's favorite hiding place. One more chirrup and out she came, trotting straight up to me with her purr in high gear. I was flattered, but after one pat on her stomach, I realized her newfound sociability had nothing to do with me. There was an unpleasant-looking bulge on the right side of her belly. She knew something was seriously wrong and had sought out human attention.

It turned out to be a simple hernia. It was repaired a few days later, and Pansy made a complete recovery, including going back to her old antisocial ways.

serious problem with your cat, that she has something that could develop into a serious problem, or even that there's anything wrong with her at all. If you catch an early warning sign, just keep a closer eye on your cat to see if the warning sign continues or worsens. Make a call to your veterinarian at your earliest convenience and discuss what you've seen. Your vet may suggest making an appointment for an exam or just ask some questions and give you some other clues to keep watch for.

Remember, any sort of behavior change may be significant, no matter how slight or unimportant it might seem. Being a good cat watcher not only helps you catch emerging health problems early—when they have the best chance of being successfully treated—it can give you a deeper appreciation for the beautiful and complex behavior of cats.

> Longhair cats don't really shed any more than shorthairs; it only appears that way since the longer hair is so visible.

Change in appearance. Does there seem to be a little less of your cat around these days? Or perhaps a little more? Assuming her diet and appetite are the same, a gain or loss of weight could be telling you something potentially more serious is happening inside your cat's body. Does her hair seem thinner? Coarser? Has it lost its healthy shine? A dull coat, excessive hair loss, or fur that feels dry, coarse, or brittle are important signs of possible health problems, too.

Of course, changes in appearance are natural with advancing age, including some loss of body bulk or somewhat scruffier-looking fur. But even these normal changes are important signals; they're saying you now have a senior citizen cat whose needs will be changing along with her body.

Changes in appetite and elimination. Cats are notorious for being picky eaters. But, in fact, finickiness isn't really a normal part of cat behavior. In general, cats will turn up their nose at food for the same three reasons kids will: It doesn't taste good; they're holding out for something better (and know they'll get it if they refuse what they've been given); or they don't feel good.

If your cat has been steadily eating the same diet, then suddenly loses enthusiasm, don't assume she's just gotten tired of the same old food. If we can eat the same breakfast cereal or have the same coffee and Danish pastry every morning, there's no reason why your cat can't be satisfied with the same menu every day. Going off her food (or, for that matter, becoming ravenously hungry) is another way your cat lets you know she's not feeling well.

Since cats use the litter box, you may not notice a change in elimination habits right away. As unpleasant as it may seem, it's a good idea to at least be aware of what you're scooping or dumping from the cat's litter. A marked increase or decrease in urine or stool, the presence of blood or mucous, or a particularly pungent smell (when the box has been recently cleaned) are all warnings of possible trouble ahead.

Likewise, a cat who is litter-box trained but suddenly seems to forget is sending you a message. It could be a behavioral, stress, or environmental thing (see Chapter 8, "Common Behavioral Problems and Home Remedies"), but it could also be triggered by worms, a bladder infection, or other potentially serious problems.

It's often hard to pinpoint if a change is strictly in behavior, appearance, or appetite and elimination. For example, pacing the floor might be considered either a behavioral change or an indication of a hyperactive thyroid gland, and a cat who has scratched off patches of hair has a change in appearance that could come from a change in behavior. What's more, changes can happen over a period of days, weeks, or months—or they can just pop up from one moment to the next.

Sudden or abrupt changes are easier to notice. Long-range changes add up over time, usually so slowly we don't catch them until they've made some significant progress. Let's go back to diabetes as an example. A cat developing diabetes will drink more and will make more frequent trips to the litter box, producing larger volumes of urine. It would be almost impossible to notice your cat making just one extra trip to the water bowl or litter box in the course of a week, and it would still be fairly difficult even when increased to an extra trip every day. And even several extra trips per day can slip past your notice, too, especially since cats are nocturnal and most of the additional water or litter-box breaks could be coming while you're asleep. By the time you're thinking, "Gee, that cat seems to be spending a lot of time at the water bowl or litter box," she's probably at the several-extra-trips-a-day level. You must work at training yourself to notice your pet's daily habits so you can detect and report any subtle and gradual changes to your vet.

KNOW WHEN TO CALL THE VET

Of course, early warnings don't do you any good if you don't do something about them. You should check out any indicators of potential health problems with your vet as soon as possible, just to make sure. But there are other times when a call to the vet—or a trip straight to the animal hospital—is a right-this-minute priority.

What Every Cat Owner Should Know

Life-Threatening Emergencies: Urinary Blockage

It strikes cats of any age, but younger adult males seem to be at the highest risk. The culprit is usually stones or sand that form in the cat's bladder, often as a result of a diet high in ash or mineral content. Once it happens, it's likely to happen again. On the plus side, when the problem occurs, there is usually an uncomplicated—but painful—way to fix it. On the negative side, it can quickly become fatal; even if the blockage is caught early, it can result in permanent damage to the cat's kidneys and other vital organs.

The urinary tract dumps the chemical wastes of everyday life out of your cat's body. If that pathway blocks up, all those wastes back up, poisoning the cat. So when a bladder stone gets lodged in the urinary tract, the clock starts ticking and every minute counts. If you notice your cat squatting in the litter box and straining or crying but not producing anything or producing small amounts of bloody urine, run—don't walk—to the nearest veterinarian.

The vet can fix the problem by "unblocking" a cat. This procedure can be as simple as a little skillful pressure and manipulation to break up the obstruction. More serious cases call for catheterization: The cat is sedated, and a flexible tube is used to clear out the blockage. In extreme cases, emergency surgery may be called for.

Any emergency situation. The common sense definition of a veterinary emergency is when you would call the doctor for yourself if it happened to you. Emergencies would therefore include:

- Profuse bleeding, including any open wound or bleeding from nose, mouth, ears, or any other body opening.

- Fractures or dislocations. If you suspect a broken bone, don't try to find the break or set it yourself. Let a professional handle it.

- Loss of consciousness.

- Fever of more than 102 degrees Fahrenheit. Cats have a normal body temperature that's a few degrees warmer than ours, but a persistent fever over 102 needs medical attention. (See the section on taking your cat's temperature in Chapter 5, "At Home Health Care: Practical Skills.")

- Difficulty breathing, swallowing, standing, or walking, including prolonged or frequent panting (cats will sometimes pant in extremely hot or humid conditions, or when they have overexerted in play), staggering, or an uncoordinated or clumsy gait. (Kittens are always a little clumsy, of course.)

- Straining or crying in the litter box, especially during urination. Some cats naturally make a big production out of using the box or even make sounds while digging, eliminating, or burying. You'll have to determine what's normal for your cat, but if you have any doubts, call the vet anyway.

- Convulsion, electrocution, or drowning.

- Blunt trauma, including high falls (see the section on high-rise syndrome in Chapter 3, "An Ounce of Prevention"), being hit by a car, or getting caught in doors or machinery, even if there is no apparent serious injury. These kinds of accidents may

What Every Cat Owner Should Know

cause internal bleeding or injuries only a veterinary exam can detect.

Any sudden significant change. While slight or gradual changes in appetite, elimination, appearance, or behavior are usually early warnings that call for timely but not necessarily immediate veterinary attention, a big or sudden shift may be cause for alarm. The chowhound cat who won't even get off the couch for breakfast one morning, for example, is showing a strong sign of potentially serious illness and needs to be checked out as soon as possible. Even if the change doesn't seem to be life-threatening, if it's a major departure from what your cat usually does, it's better to invest a little time and money and find out it's nothing than to take a "wait-and-see" approach and find out it's really something serious but it's also too late to do anything about it.

Any symptom that persists more than 48 hours or worsens (even a relatively mild one). Let's say you notice your cat has started sneezing a lot. It could be that she just crawled into a dusty nook somewhere, or it could be the start of a feline cold. If the sneezing doesn't go away after several hours, the cold begins to look like the more likely choice. If your cat is still sneezing a lot by the second day, it's pretty clear it's not going away by itself any time soon and it's time to call the vet.

Of course, if any symptom worsens suddenly or interferes with your cat's breathing, eating, drinking, walking, or elimination, don't wait 48 hours. Call the vet immediately.

Can I Catch It From My Cat?: Zoonotic Diseases

A lot of city folk have the notion that animals carry all kinds of dangerous diseases. Some of those fears are well founded, especially among wild or exotic animals. But the truth is, there aren't very many serious diseases you can catch from a domestic animal—and especially not from a pet. Otherwise, it wouldn't make sense that they'd be pets.

Before we go any further, there are a few myths to put to rest. There are a couple of cat diseases that have names that sound a little too close to some very serious human diseases for comfort. Feline leukemia virus (FeLV) does cause leukemia . . . in cats and in cats only. FeLV does not cause leukemia in people, and it can't even live in the human body. There's no danger that a FeLV-positive cat is going to make her owner sick.

Feline immunodeficiency virus (FIV) sounds a lot like the human immunodeficiency virus (HIV), the virus associated with AIDS. That's no coincidence: FIV and HIV belong to the same class of viruses, but that's where the similarities end. FIV does not infect people and can not cause human AIDS. Some folks—and even some vets—call FIV "feline AIDS" as a quick way of describing what the virus does. Unfortunately, the name just adds to the confusion. AIDS is a human disease, and FIV is a cat disease.

There's also virtually no chance that your cat's cold will get passed to you—or, for that matter, that your cold will get passed to her. The viruses that usually cause sneezing, coughing, and runny nose and eyes in cats don't infect people.

Cats can get some of the same diseases that people also get: diabetes, arthritis, heart disease, and cancer, to mention a few. But since none of these diseases are contagious, there's no way you can catch them from your cat.

Generally, cats are thought of as being less dangerous than dogs (you don't see any front-page stories about a vicious Siamese that bit the arm off some poor delivery person), and their reputation for cleanliness give the impression that they carry no diseases at all. But in fact, most vets would rather face an angry dog than an angry cat. (Cats can slash you with all four feet and bite.) And there are a few things you can catch from your cat. Here are some of the human-cat diseases you should know about.

Fleas. These hardy little insects bite warm-blooded animals and use their blood for food. Fleas are so tiny that a single bite is barely noticeable (unless you or your cat are allergic, in which case it itches like crazy). A full-blown flea infestation, however, can take so much blood from an animal that it becomes anemic.

Fortunately for us, fleas prefer the warmer body temperature of cats and dogs to our 98.6 degrees Fahrenheit. But a hungry flea will take any port in a storm, and a flea will jump from an infected cat to carpets, drapes, furniture, and later onto you for a quick snack.

There's some concern that diseases carried in the blood could be passed through fleas but that would mean the flea that bites you would have to have bitten another person with a blood-borne disease, which is possible but not highly likely. The largest dangers of fleas are the annoyance and itching of the bites.

Ticks. These are also blood-sucking insects. Ticks are somewhat larger than fleas, especially once they've attached themselves to a host and swell up. Like fleas, ticks aren't as likely to abandon your cat for you, but it can happen. Also, if your cat has been somewhere that ticks hang out, the odds are either you've been there, too, or your cat has brought them home. Again, the most common problem is annoyance. However, ticks can carry two serious diseases: Rocky mountain spotted fever and Lyme disease.

The best protection against both of these diseases is prompt and complete removal of ticks. A few generations of Boy Scouts were taught that the best way to remove a tick is to burn its fanny with a cigarette or a smouldering match head. Well, besides the fact that Boy Scouts shouldn't be smoking, the evict-a-tick-by-fire strategy is not the best choice.

The best way to remove a tick is to use a pair of tweezers to grasp the tick as close to the skin line as possible. Pull it straight out, firmly but gently, with slow, even pressure. This should remove the entire tick—including the head. Ticks are very hardy, so drop it in a small bottle of rubbing alcohol to make sure it's dead (and to preserve it for your vet, if your cat shows any signs of illness). Then, once you have removed the tick, dab the area with a topical antiseptic or antibiotic ointment.

Worms. These little fellows can live in your digestive tract without you realizing they've taken up residence. Worms can be picked up by careless handling of litter boxes and soil that cats have used as a litter box. Children are at particular risk for picking up worms this way.

Worms are often hard to detect, since they live inside the body. The tip-off is usually some sort of digestive problem that doesn't go away and has no other explanation. It's also a good idea to take a sample of your pet's stool to the vet for microscopic examination of worms and worm eggs. Worms can be treated quickly and safely as soon as they are diagnosed.

Ringworm. This isn't really a worm at all. It's a fungus that takes up residence on the skin, causing bald, scaly patches that are usually edged by a red ring. Cats are notorious for being asymptomatic carriers of ringworm, which simply means they can carry the fungus into your home (and onto you) without ever showing any signs themselves. Of course, many cats do show the signs, too.

Whether your cat shows the signs or you do (or both of you do), you'll most likely have to treat the whole house, as well as all the cats in the home. Ringworm spores can survive in the nooks and crannies

CATS AND PREGNANCY: THE STRAIGHT STORY

One of the most common—and saddest—bits of misinformation that gets handed out about cats is that cats and pregnancy don't mix. While it's true that toxoplasmosis can cause serious birth defects, that's primarily true for a woman who is infected with toxoplasmosis for the first time during her first trimester of pregnancy. Infection for the first time during the second and third trimester can cause some problems, but they are rare.

A simple blood test can determine if a woman has already been exposed to the toxoplasma organism. If she has, she's immune and it's nearly impossible that toxoplasmosis will be of any concern. If not, she should just take precautions to prevent infection: Never clean the litter box, wear gloves when gardening or working with plants and wash hands thoroughly afterward, and avoid eating raw or undercooked meat. She should also take extreme care handling meat, making sure not to touch her mouth or nose and washing thoroughly immediately afterward. It is not necessary to remove cats from the home of a pregnant woman.

of your home for months. Treatments might include disinfecting your home, topical ointments or lotions for the scaly patches, dips or baths for your cat, and oral medication.

Rabies. This is serious business. Rabies is a fatal disease. What's more, once the disease has taken hold, there's not much that can be done to stop it. The best defense against rabies is a strong offense. An indoor cat has nearly no chance of being exposed to rabies, but the safest bet is to give your cat a rabies vaccine and keep it current. Rabies is passed in the bite or scratch of an infected animal, so every time an outdoor cat gets in a scrape with another cat or tangles with local wildlife, there's a chance she'll contract it.

Rabies infects all warm-blooded animals, including people. Any bite or scratch from an animal—even one that you know and that's up-to-date with its rabies shots—should be treated as potentially dangerous. It's never an overreaction to seek medical care for a cat bite or serious cat scratch.

Cat scratch disease (also referred to as cat scratch fever). Some folks insist that cat scratch fever is a myth, but it really is a medically proven disease. Cat scratches and bites can turn into serious infections literally overnight. Cat bites, in particular, need careful attention. Wash bites or serious scratches thoroughly and call your doctor for advice. You may need a tetanus booster or an antibiotic shot to prevent infection.

Toxoplasmosis. Toxoplasma gondii is a protozoan parasite (one-celled organism) that can cause a neurologic disease in humans. This protozoa is passed in the stools of infected cats, who in turn catch it from infected animals they've killed and eaten. Cats are what's called the primary vector for the toxoplasma organism, which means the life cycle of the parasite depends on spending at least a little time in the body of a cat.

What Every Cat Owner Should Know

Cats don't usually show much in the way of symptoms when they're infected with toxoplasmosis—and a person who picks it up usually doesn't either. There may be some mild symptoms that are passed off as a cold or the flu but that's usually about it. The two major exceptions are people whose immune systems are weakened (such as someone on chemotherapy or a person with AIDS) and pregnant women.

Perhaps as many as 70 percent of adults have already been infected by toxoplasmosis and are now immune. Although cats are the primary vector for this parasite—and it is theoretically possible to pick up toxoplasmosis from careless handling of litter boxes or inhaling toxoplasma spores when cleaning the litter box—most people get toxoplasmosis from digging in dirt contaminated by cat feces or handling or eating raw or undercooked meat.

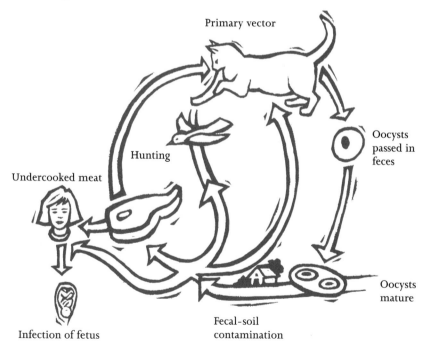

Primary vector

Hunting

Undercooked meat

Oocysts passed in feces

Oocysts mature

Infection of fetus

Fecal-soil contamination

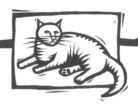

At-Home Health Care: Practical Skills

Give a man a fish—he eats for a day;
Teach a man to fish—he eats for a lifetime.

. . . to which my old pal, Hoke Mitchell, likes to add: "Give a cat a fish—and he'll come back the next day looking for another one."

Hoke's dubious sense of humor aside, the point here is that having some basic at-home health care skills can be a lifesaver—for your cat's life, that is. And it's best to learn those skills right now; an emergency is no time to start learning feline first aid or the right way to handle and move a sick or injured cat.

How Sick Is My Cat?: Evaluating Your Cat's Condition at Home

Your cat can actually tell you a lot about how he's feeling, if you can understand what he's saying. No, there's no secret code to your cat's meows and purrs. But in many ways you might otherwise overlook, your cat is making clear statements about his health. Here's what to look for and what to do.

Behavior. Vets get a lot of the same kinds of phone calls. One of the most common is what the staff at one animal hospital has dubbed a "comedian cat" call. That's when the owner calls and says, "My cat is acting funny..."

Many times a cat will "act funny" at home, but he'll be so nervous at the vet's office, he won't do anything; so the more accurate your report, the better your vet can determine what's going on. And since describing your cat's condition as "funny" or "sick" is a little too vague to pin a solid diagnosis on, you need to specifically describe what your cat is doing. A good idea is to write out a detailed description of what you see. (It's not a good idea to take time to do this in a life-threatening emergency, of course.) Try to think of the way you would try to describe to your doctor an ailment or pain you're experiencing. Some descriptions seem easy such as "My cat is coughing" but might be a little trickier than you think. What you call coughing, another cat owner might call choking. Paint a picture of what you see with words, even imitating the sound, if you can.

Appetite and elimination. As unpleasant as it may seem, keeping a close eye on what goes into and out of your cat's body is a valuable home health care tool. How much food a cat needs will depend a lot on his age, life stage (growth, pregnancy, lactation, or old age, for example), activity, and the type of food he gets. How much he eats is more a function of how much food is available and his health.

If you notice your cat isn't eating as much as before, you also need to know the context. For example, does he just seem uninterested in food? Or does he come running as usual for his food but then eats little (if any) of it? In the first case, it would be completely correct to

DIRTY WORK: COLLECTING URINE AND STOOL SAMPLES FOR THE VET

One of the best ways to check out what's going on inside a cat is to analyze what comes out of him. Problems as routine as worms or as serious as diabetes and kidney disease can be caught by checking stool or urine samples. A cat can be hospitalized and the animal hospital staff can collect the samples, but it's a lot of stress on the cat, and some cats will just hold it while they're in a strange place. So when a stool or urine sample is called for, it's usually up to you to get it.

Here's an easy trick for collecting either kind of sample. Close your cat in a room with his own litter box. The box should be thoroughly washed first and filled with those plastic foam "peanuts" used for packing. (If those aren't available, you can try cut-up plastic trash bags instead.) Listen for your cat to start scratching in the box and collect samples as quickly as possible. (If a cat urinates and defecates in the box, the urine sample is contaminated and can't be used.)

Collect urine samples in a clean, dry container with a tight-fitting lid. Stool samples can be collected in an ordinary sandwich bag and sealed with a twist-tie. Samples should be taken straight to the vet. If you can't leave immediately, they can be refrigerated for up to three hours.

say your cat has no appetite; he isn't hungry. In the second case, he's definitely interested in food; he has an appetite but something is making him feel like he can't eat very much.

It's usually not polite to talk about elimination, and most of us aren't comfortable discussing it in the kind of detail that you need to know to help a sick cat. But it is important in understanding the health of your cat. Are stools well formed, soft, or loose? Is there any trace of blood in urine or feces? Is there mucus in the stool? Even things like color or odor can be important.

Of course, eating and elimination are two sides of the same coin (or two ends of the same digestive system, to be more accurate), so pay attention to how they go together. For example, if your cat has a ravenous appetite but doesn't seem to put on any weight (or actually seems thinner), that should alert you to a possible problem. He could be the feline equivalent of those people we all envy who can eat anything and never gain an ounce—or there could be something a little more serious going on. Once you've noticed these changes in your cat, take him to the vet to determine the cause of the problem.

Mucus membranes. This is the term for the skin that lines the mouth and nose. It's pretty tough to look up a cat's nose, so that's probably out of the question. You might be able to get your cat to cooperate with looking in his mouth for a second, but the odds are he won't be too pleased. Still, how to open a reluctant cat's mouth is something every cat owner should know.

The best way to check your cat's mouth is to grasp the top of your cat's head with your thumb on one side and your fingers on the other. Tip your cat's head back so his nose points upward. Now, using your other hand, put one finger where the front teeth meet and push down gently with steady pressure on the lower jaw. As your cat's mouth opens, you'll have a few seconds to get a good look inside.

The color of the skin in your cat's mouth and on his gums tell an important story. A healthy cat usually has a tinge of pink. Stark white could be a sign of anemia. A yellow-ish cast (jaundice) is often a sign of liver trouble. A bluish tint may mean your cat isn't taking up enough oxygen, usually a result of a respiratory problem or poisoning.

> A typical cat can have 130,000 hairs per square inch on his belly.

If your cat isn't cooperating with having his mouth opened—or you're squeamish about doing it—you can also check the color of his gums. Hold his head the same way you would to open his mouth. Gently pull down on the skin covering the lower teeth at the corner of the mouth, using the thumb and forefinger of your other hand.

A word of warning, though. It's not unusual for a cat's gums—and even the roof of his mouth—to take on some of his coat color, especially as he gets older. For some reason, orange cats are also prone to developing "freckles" on their lips, gums, and inside their mouths. Black gums on a black cat aren't anything to worry about, but pale, yellowish, or bluish tinged gums on any cat should be reported to your veternarian right away.

Coat condition. A healthy, well-groomed cat has a soft, clean, slightly lustrous coat. A cat whose fur is dull, dry, oily, or unkempt may not be getting groomed well enough or often enough by his owner, or he may be under the weather.

Even with regular grooming by humans, a cat needs to do some of his own grooming to keep his coat looking good. Cats are usually pretty diligent about their personal hygiene, so a cat who's not keeping up his appearance is likely not being lazy, he doesn't feel good.

On the other hand, a cat who's grooming himself raw is also telling you something. Excessive grooming can be a sign of stress, a skin problem, or a reaction to fleas. Look for "hot spots"—patches where your cat licks so much that the fur is gone and the skin is red or raw.

Of course, not all hair loss is from grooming. Take note of any bald patches or areas where the hair is thin or sparse. Most of your cat's body should be covered with a coat of hair thick enough to hide the skin underneath. (About the only place where it's normal for the fur to be thinned out is the area between your cat's eyes and ears.) Whatever the case, your vet's advice will help put your cat back on the path to a healthy coat.

Ears. Make it a point to check your cat's ears periodically. Grooming time is a good time to do this. Look for a change in color inside the ears. Just like the gums and inside of the mouth, a yellowish or bluish cast to the skin on the inside of your cat's ears can be a sign of a major health problem; alert your veterinarian right away.

Cats do a pretty good job of keeping their ears clean. Outside of some normal wax, then, you shouldn't see much in your cat's ears other than . . . well, ear. Any sort of inflammation, raw skin, or crustiness is a tip that something's amiss. Debris in a cat's ear—it usually looks like dirt or coffee grounds—is an indication of ear mites, tiny insects that live and breed in the ear canal. Itchiness is another sign of ear mites, but not all cats with ear mites will scratch or rub at their ears—and not all cats who scratch or rub their ears have ear mites.

Cats who go outdoors need to have their ears inspected from time to time for other reasons. In cold weather, frostbite is a real danger. Those nice, tall, pointy feline ears are made up mostly of skin and cartilage. There isn't a lot of blood flow to the ears. Even being caught

CPR for Cats

A cat who stops breathing needs mouth-to-mouth resuscitation. A cat whose heart and breathing stop needs cardiopulmonary resuscitation (CPR). If you think your cat needs mouth-to-mouth or CPR, he also needs to get to the vet as soon as possible. Call for help, get a friend to start driving you to the animal hospital, or call a cab—before you do anything else.

Be sure the cat really needs resuscitation. Giving mouth-to-mouth or CPR to a cat who doesn't need it (or practicing them on a healthy cat) can do serious harm.

If the cat is:

• Breathing; heartbeat present (feel for it by gently grasping the cat's chest, thumb and fore-fingers on either side of the rib cage just below the armpits): Do not begin mouth-to-mouth or CPR.

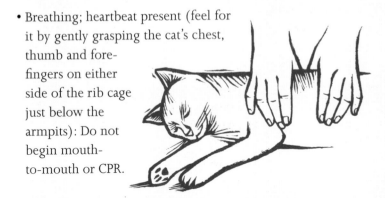

outside for an hour when the temperature takes a sudden drop can be enough for the tips of your cat's ears to freeze.

Outdoor (or indoor/outdoor) cats are also more likely to get into scrapes with other cats. The ears are easy targets for scratches and

At-Home Health Care: Practical Skills

- Not breathing; heartbeat present: Begin mouth-to-mouth resuscitation. Grasp the cat's muzzle with one hand, cover his nose and mouth with your mouth, blow gently, then remove your mouth to let him exhale; repeat about 12 times per minute.

- Not breathing, no heartbeat felt, bluish cast to the tongue or inside of the mouth: Begin CPR immediately.

To begin CPR, grasp the cat's chest as you check for heartbeat and gently compress the ribcage on a three-count sequence—squeeze for two counts, release on three— about 80 to 100 times a minute. Continue giving mouth-to-mouth. If you have help, your part- ner should give one breath after every five compressions, making sure not to give a breath until you have released the last compression. If you're working alone, give two breaths after every 15 compressions.

bites during even the mildest of cat fights. A cat's small, sharp teeth can make a puncture wound that seals up immediately, trapping dirt and germs inside, causing infection. The cat may look and act alright when he comes home, but a few days later an abscess—a tender, swollen area of trapped pus—may form, and the cat can run a fever. At this point, you'll need to take your cat to the vet.

Eyes. "The eyes," goes the old saying, "are the windows of the soul." Fortunately for cat owners, the eyes are also a window to how your cat is feeling.

- A cat's pupils can look like anything from vertical slits, to the classic spindle-shaped "cat's eye," to full dilation—big black dots that take up all of the colored part of the eye. Certain diseases, including trouble in a cat's nervous system, can cause the pupils to be noticeably different sizes. A cloudy, milky, or filmy look to the pupils might be a sign of cataracts, viral ulcers, or other vision problems.

- The iris is the colored part of the eye. Cats usually have some variety of green, yellow, or blue eyes. Occasionally, a cat will be "odd-eyed"; each eye is a different color. If you notice changes in your cat's iris or the appearance of splotches of other colors, contact your vet. (Note: It's not unusual for the iris to change with age. Old cats' irises may take on a "Swiss cheese" look, as if they're falling apart—although they aren't!)

> People in China used to believe that the size of a cat's pupils could tell the height of the sun.

- The "white" of the eye is known officially as the sclera. Obviously, this should be white (perhaps with some small blood vessels visible). Yellow or "bloodshot" sclera, ulcers or splotches of color, and signs of damage (like scrapes or bruises) are indicators of trouble.

At-Home Health Care: Practical Skills

Taking Your Cat's Temperature

You can't really rely on touching your cat to tell if he's running a fever, and you can't get him to hold a thermometer under his tongue. However, there are other options for taking a cat's temperature: under the armpit and in the ear canal. The first of these isn't very reliable, and the second requires an expensive electronic thermometer. Unfortunately, the most accurate and reliable way to take your cat's temperature is the way he's going to like least—rectally.

Obviously, a rectal thermometer is the equipment called for here. Shake the thermometer down below 99 degrees Fahrenheit, and lubricate the end with petroleum jelly or vegetable oil. With his feet firmly planted on a secure surface, tuck your cat under one arm with his tail pointed outward and his nose back by your elbow. With the hand of that same arm, hold the cat's tail up, and gently insert the thermometer in the anus with the other hand (you may have to bear down slightly at first). Slowly insert the thermometer about one inch, and keep it there for up to three minutes, if possible. Gently remove the thermometer, wipe off the glass, and read the temperature.

- Conjunctiva is the pink, fleshy stuff under the eyelids that helps hold the eye in place. You usually don't notice the conjunctiva unless it swells up, in which case it may protrude from under the eyelid, giving the eye a "meaty" appearance.

- The third eyelid appears when your cat blinks or closes his eyes; this wonderful adaptation moves from the inside corner of the eye to cover the front surface of the eyeball. Again, it's something you rarely notice unless there's a problem. One of the ways cats announce that they don't feel well is when their third eyelids are up—that is, they've moved partially across the eyeball.

Hydration. A cat who hasn't been eating well may also not be drinking enough to meet all of his needs for water, and he may become dehydrated. To check your cat's hydration, gently grasp the skin between his shoulder blades, pull up slightly, and open your fingers to let go. If the skin snaps back into place immediately, your cat is well hydrated. If not, the odds are the cat is dehydrated and may need to be rehydrated by your veterinarian to prevent serious harm.

Coughing, sneezing, runny nose and eyes. An occasional cough or sneeze—or even an occasional bout of coughing or sneezing—is a normal reaction to the millions of unseen irritants in the air. Even good, clean country air has pollen, dust, and other tiny things floating around in it. So if your cat sneezes or coughs now and then, it's probably nothing to worry about.

Of course, cats are notorious for coughing up hairballs—another natural part of being a cat (especially a longhair cat). Regular grooming can keep down the number and severity of these clumps of swallowed fur (some well-groomed shorthair cats never seem to get them), but periodic coughing or "throat-clearing" sounds are also pretty normal.

Repeated or frequent bouts of sneezing or coughing are usually a sign of a health problem. Sneezing accompanied by a "runny nose" is a definite symptom of illness, as is swelling or discharge from your cat's eyes.

Temperature. Ever notice that a cat is particularly nice to cuddle up to on a chilly night? That's because the average body temperature for a cat is about 101.4 degrees Farhenheit (a good three degrees warmer

> Cats love heat, and their bodies won't feel discomfort until their skin temperature reaches about 126 degrees Fahrenheit.

than ours), although an individual cat's temperature may range between 100 and 102.5 degrees Farhenheit and still be considered "normal." Disease—or prolonged exposure to heat or cold—can send a cat's temperature above or below the normal range.

Usually, a mild fever is a normal part of a cat's natural disease-fighting system. But extremely high or persistent fever can do serious—or even fatal—damage, and calls for professional help.

HANDLING, RESTRAINING, AND MOVING A SICK OR INJURED CAT

If you think you know some people who make difficult patients when they're sick, at least those folks aren't likely to bite and scratch you to the point that you need medical attention. A sick or injured cat is scared and in pain, and, therefore, likely to be very touchy and defensive.

You have to give a cat like that some healthy respect: Those teeth and claws can do some serious damage. But it's just as important to know how to handle and hold your cat with confidence in an emergency. In fact, you're less likely to get hurt if you have a good technique and act decisively.

A really sick cat may be fairly easy to handle and move if he's weak or lethargic from his illness. To transport a seriously ill cat—or any cat, for that matter—use a sturdy carrier with enough bedding to keep him warm and comfortable. The carrier shouldn't be too big or else the cat will get jostled. Be sure you keep checking on a cat who's

The Home Veterinary First Aid Kit

You can buy a ready-made kit or put one together yourself. Here are some useful items to have on hand.

- Disinfectants/antiseptics:

    povidone-iodine (0.001 percent to 1 percent dilution)

    hydrogen peroxide (not stronger than 3 percent solution)

    dilute Dakin's solution (one part household bleach to 20 parts water)

- Bulb syringe or turkey baster (for flushing wounds)

- Cotton swabs

- Gauze bandages, tape, bandage scissors

- Socks (for bandages and splints)

- Splints

- Cotton balls

- Rectal thermometer, petroleum jelly

- Tweezers and forceps (for removing ticks and foreign bodies)

It's also a good idea to include your vet's phone number, the animal emergency hospital phone number, and a first aid handbook in the kit.

unconscious or not moving a lot, making sure his breathing and other vital signs are okay.

Moving an injured cat is a lot trickier. Try to splint or otherwise immobilize broken or crushed limbs, and keep the cat reclining as much as possible. Again, a cozy-size carrier with comfortable bedding will help. Even healthy cats will fight going into a carrier head-first, so try setting the carrier on its back end and lowering the cat tail first. Close the door quickly; then gently tip the carrier down to its regular position.

For a cat who is struggling wildly, don't press the fight—you'll only get hurt, and the cat will get hurt worse than he already is. Pop the cat into a pillow case and tie an overhand knot in the open end. The weave of the fabric allows air through, and the complete enclosure is actually reassuring for the cat.

There are several occasions where you may have to restrain your cat: for examination, treatment, medication, grooming, or just to carry him. Here are some tried-and-true techniques for restraining cats.

The "Press." With one hand, grasp the scruff of the cat's neck. Place the palm of the other hand over the cat's sacrum (the "lower back," just above the tail), and press down with firm, gentle pressure with both hands. This is a low-level restraint technique, for a relatively calm cat.

Football hold. This is a common one. With the cat's body resting on a solid surface, tuck him under one arm like a football, using your elbow to snuggle his body up against your side. Grasp his forelegs between the fingers of the hand of the restraining arm. Your other hand is free to do whatever has to be done or to grasp the cat's scruff if more secure restraint is needed for someone else to do something to him.

Throw in the towel. If you need to get to the cat's mouth or face (such as to give pills, liquid medicine, eye ointment, or ear mite medication), you can wrap up the rest of the cat in a thick towel. A good swaddling, leaving just the head out, will keep those claws under wraps and probably reduce struggling. Use the football hold on a wrapped-up cat.

GIVING CATS MEDICATIONS

Mary Poppins can sing about "a spoonful of sugar" until the cows come home, but nothing is going to convince a cat to take his medicine willingly. A notable exception was an old cat named Buddy, who would eat just about anything that didn't eat him first. About one day out of three, you could get him to take his thyroid medicine just by dropping the pill on the floor in front of him—he'd gulp it down before he realized what it was. But not all cats are like Buddy, so here are some ways to get your cat to take his medicine.

Liquid medicines are administered with an eye dropper or syringe. Open the cat's mouth and squirt the liquid slowly into the back of his throat. You can also slip the end of the dropper or syringe between the back teeth and squirt the liquid into the back of the throat that way. Hold the cat's head steady and keep his nose pointing up until everything is swallowed, otherwise he might shake his head and send the medication flying around the room instead. Gently rub the cat's throat to stimulate swallowing.

To give your cat a pill, open his mouth using the technique described for checking mucous membranes. There's one important variation, though: Hold the pill or capsule to be given between your thumb and forefinger, and use the middle finger of the same hand to lever open the lower jaw. Place the pill at the back of the cat's mouth, in the groove at the base of the tongue. You may have to nudge the pill slightly with your index finger to trigger the swallowing reflex. You can also try blowing gently on the cat's nose, or running your finger across it. If the cat licks his nose, he's probably swallowed the pill.

For cats who have an especially hard time taking pills, you can try crushing the tablet and mixing it in with his favorite snack. Most cats can detect even the slightest "doctoring" of their food, but it's worth a try when other methods fail.

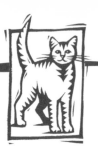

COMMON PHYSICAL PROBLEMS AND HOME REMEDIES

So now we come to the "meat and potatoes" of this book. Everything you've read until now is like setting the table for a dinner party. Think about it: Cooking a gourmet six-course meal won't do you much more good than fast food if you don't serve it right. Likewise, the information in chapters 1 through 5 is absolutely necessary to make these remedies work right.

The physical problems in this chapter run the range from A to Z (well, actually from Asthma to Worms). Many of the entries have a "When to Call the Vet" section, too. Be sure to read this carefully since there's only so much you can do at home.

Asthma

What it is

Asthma is a chronic breathing problem. Both cats and people suffer from it, but it isn't contagious. An asthmatic cat (or person) has bouts of extremely difficult breathing called asthma attacks. An asthma attack is fairly easy to spot; you'll notice rapid, open-mouthed breathing accompanied by wheezing and often by forced exhalations. Because breathing is so severely restricted during an asthma attack, the cat's gums and tongue may take on a bluish color. (Do not try to give mouth-to-mouth resuscitation or CPR to a cat having an asthma attack.)

Asthma often develops from another breathing problem called allergic bronchitis. This is pretty much what it sounds like: The airways in the cat's lungs get inflamed as the result of an allergic reaction to inhaled germs, dust (including dust from litter), wood smoke, and other irritants. Usually the cat has no other major signs of illness, a normal temperature, and continues to eat well. The only telltale sign is that she just has fits of deep, moist-sounding coughing. If the allergic bronchitis goes untreated or the source of the allergy isn't removed, the lungs can be permanently damaged, resulting in emphysema and asthma. Once the damage is done, even removing the original cause or causes of the allergic bronchitis won't make asthma go away.

Recently, some studies have been done on the effects of secondhand smoke on pets. The news is about what you'd expect: Secondhand smoke isn't particularly good for your cat. Cats with asthma or other breathing problems suffer more from secondhand smoke. Remember, asthma is related to allergies, so anything that irritates the air passages of the lungs—including cigarette smoke—can trigger an asthma attack.

Reduce stress. Stress makes allergies and asthma worse. Right about now you're saying to yourself, "Stress? What the heck kind of stress does a cat have?" That's a fair question. They certainly don't have to worry about paying bills or where their next meal is coming from. (Those are your stresses, actually.) They don't have job pressures or deadlines to meet. Heck, they don't even have to think about what they're going to wear every day.

> Your cat helps keep you healthy—the simple act of petting your cat reduces stress and lowers blood pressure.

Cats have stress that we like to call "domestication stress" or "family stress." You see, cats weren't originally designed and built to live among humans. They've done a superb job of adapting, but no matter how independent and primal your cat seems, she's still having to deal with the human world and human civilization every single day. And that gets tough. Giving her plenty of options to do cat things such as run, climb, stalk (preferably another cat), bat things around, hide, and nap in secluded spots helps her cope.

If the stress level goes up in your life or in your household, it goes up in your cat's life, too. She can't understand why things are getting tense—she just knows people are moving and sounding anxious. Remember, "stress" doesn't just mean negative things; positive events carry stress, too. In fact, probably the worst kind of stress for a cat is change. A new baby, for instance, is not only a time for great joy but also for great change—and the stresses that go with that. For you, those stresses mean less sleep (or none at all), a change in lifestyle, and an extra mouth to feed. For your cat, it means some strange new animal, who makes odd noises, smells funny, and doesn't do much, suddenly takes all the human attention away from her!

Clear the air. Secondhand smoke isn't the only thing that can make asthma worse. Even things that we think make our home more pleasant can be a no-no for a cat with bronchitis or asthma. Perfumes, room fresheners, deodorizers, and even scented litters or litter additives can trigger allergy and asthma attacks. Likewise, the fumes from paints, cleaners, varnishes, and new carpeting are actually chemical irritants that create problems for the asthmatic cat. Use natural objects, such as flowers, eucalyptus sprigs, and fresh floral potpourri, to provide a fresh scent to a room instead of sprays or solids that contain chemicals. Use strong-smelling paints, stains, cleaners, and solvents in well-ventilated rooms, and keep the cat out until the smell goes away. And put out those smokes.

It's a good idea to use plain, natural, unscented litter (see the section on litter box accidents in Chapter 8, "Common Behavioral Problems and Home Remedies") and to stay away from deodorizers you add to the litter. Also the dust from the litter itself irritates the lungs and can cause attacks in asthmatic cats. Some natural litters—like the ones made of recycled paper—have virtually no dust at all. To cut down on dust from clay litters, pour them slowly, keeping the opening of the bag just a few inches from the litter box.

Wetter is better. Dry air dries out the lining of your cat's air passages, encouraging coughing and making your cat more vulnerable to infection and allergic reactions. Be sure to have a good humidifier going, especially in winter, during heating season, and in arid areas of the country. There's an added bonus to this remedy: You will also be less likely to have as many coughs, stuffy noses, and colds in the air if your home is kept properly moist.

Moderation in all things. A sedentary cat is more prone to health problems, but a cat who already has asthma can have a severe attack if she exerts herself too much. On the other hand, if she barely exerts at all, her breathing will be more labored because her heart and lungs aren't fit. Plus, she'll probably gain weight, and the heavier the cat, the more trouble she'll have with her asthma. Stick to the right amount of a high-quality, healthy diet; cut out the snacks and treats; and make sure your cat stays active. Get her a feline playmate and a good supply of toys. Be certain to play with her yourself, but keep the play sessions short and low-impact.

☎ WHEN TO CALL THE VET

Any full-blown asthma attack is a medical emergency, which means your cat needs immediate veterinary medical care. Likewise, if your cat gasps for air, collapses, or turns blue in the gums and tongue, don't wait to take her to the animal hospital. Milder signs (such as noisy breath, occasional and intermittent wheezing or moist coughs, or slightly labored breathing after exertion) aren't emergencies, but you should get your cat to the vet as soon as possible. They could be caused by something other than allergies. And if it is bronchitis or the start of asthma, your vet may be able to give your cat medication that can prevent the danger and fright of a full-blown attack.

✳ DANGER LEVEL: Dangerous; a severe asthma attack can be fatal.

COUGHING

WHAT IT IS

We all know what coughing is and that it has different sounds: a dry, hacking cough; a moist-sounding cough; a single, gagging cough; a wheezing cough; and that half-cough, half-clearing the throat thing. Coughing is a reflex; when something irritates the back of the throat, breathing passages, or lungs, the body responds, expelling whatever is causing the irritation. But coughing is one of those reflexes that is not completely beyond conscious control; when needed, it can be done at will. In other words, coughing is an important mechanism for protecting the lungs and air passages from foreign objects and expelling infectious matter from the body.

WHAT TO DO ABOUT IT

From hairballs to heart trouble there are many reasons why a cat might cough. For a cat with any kind of cough or respiratory trouble, follow the steps for helping a cat with asthma. Other kinds of help depend on why the cat is coughing.

Hairballs are a common problem of cats and can be easily treated (see the section on hairballs in this chapter). Persistent coughs due to feline colds or flu can sometimes be helped with over-the-counter cough suppressants. (Do not use any cough medicine or other over-the-counter drug without the advice of your veterinarian. And keep in mind that dosages will vary widely.) If your cat is coughing and also pawing at her mouth or shaking her head, there may be something stuck in her throat or mouth. Open your cat's mouth—taking care that you avoid being bitten—and look inside. If you find a foreign body and can remove it easily, go ahead. Then keep a close eye on your cat for the next few days to see if infection develops. If, however, the object is stuck in the roof of the mouth, between the teeth, or you can't locate it, see your vet right away.

A collar can sometimes be the cause of a cough, especially if it's too tight. If your cat wears a collar, check the size. You should be able to slip the tip of your finger between the collar and the cat's neck easily. Since cats like to squeeze into tight places, collars can pose a choking hazard. Many experts recommend you only use cat collars with elastic or breakaway features so that if the cat gets the collar snagged, it comes off easily.

Any cough that persists for more than 24 hours or is accompanied by wheezing, shortness of breath, or bluish gums and tongue means a trip to the vet. Coughs combined with other serious symptoms should prompt a call to the vet, too.

✳ DANGER LEVEL: Coughs by themselves are signs of something else; they may be annoying but are usually not dangerous. Keep in mind, however, a cough may be a sign of a serious or dangerous condition.

CYSTITIS (BLADDER INFLAMMATION)

WHAT IT IS

A cat's bladder can become inflamed because of infection or irritation. Cystitis most often happens as part of a collection of bladder and urinary problems commonly called feline urological syndrome (FUS) or feline lower urinary tract disease (FLUTD). Attacks of cystitis or FUS (which includes cystitis, along with inflammation of the urinary tract and the forma-

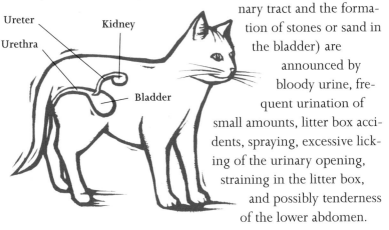

tion of stones or sand in the bladder) are announced by bloody urine, frequent urination of small amounts, litter box accidents, spraying, excessive licking of the urinary opening, straining in the litter box, and possibly tenderness of the lower abdomen.

The pH of a cat's urine—how acidic or alkaline it is—has a lot to do with cystitis and FUS. If the cat's urine is alkaline, it's much easier for urinary crystals to form. These crystals in turn form a gritty "sand" or small stones that irritate the lining of the bladder and can plug up the urinary opening in male cats, which is an extremely serious problem.

WHAT TO DO ABOUT IT

Serious complications of cystitis and FUS show up most often in adult male cats. The first flare-up usually occurs when the cat is fairly young, and repeat bouts can pop up for the rest of his life. That having been said, don't think that just because you have an older or female cat that you're in the clear: Urinary tract problems can strike any cat.

Food for thought. Although there's still some discussion about this, most experts agree that diet is a major factor in feline bladder problems. Plant-based cat foods tend to make a cat's urine more alkaline (higher pH), which encourages the formation of crystals and stones and is a more hospitable environment for bacteria. Some commercial dry cat foods seem to have the same effect on urinary pH. As a result, cats who develop cystitis or FUS should only eat dry foods recommended by a veterinarian or stick to prescription dry food specially formulated for cats with bladder problems. Your vet may also suggest a urinary acidifier to add to your cat's diet, making sure the pH of his urine stays low enough to prevent bladder stones.

Magnesium is an important trace nutrient that every cat needs. Unfortunately, some commercial cat foods provide it in a form that also encourages crystals to form in the cat's urine, which can lead to bladder stones and which, in turn, can cause a urinary obstruction. A quality commercial canned food is usually relatively low in magnesium, easy to digest, produces more acidic urine, and provides more fluid intake.

Water, water everywhere. The body is an amazing thing: If it doesn't have enough of something it needs, it finds a way to get it. If a cat isn't drinking enough, his body will find a way to conserve and reclaim water. One way is by reabsorbing water from the urine, making it more concentrated. The urinary tract lining in cats that have already had a bout of cystitis or FUS is particularly sensitive, and concentrated urine can trigger additional attacks.

Make sure your cat has constant access to plenty of clean, fresh water. Watch for your cat's drinking preferences—some favor a water faucet or even the toilet over a water bowl on the floor. It might seem odd or even a little bit disgusting, but it's probably a good idea to cater to his water-drinking whims, especially if the option is a flare-up of bladder disease.

Cats also get water from their food. The higher the moisture content in his diet, the more water he's getting—even without drinking. A cat who eats canned food gets a lot of water with the meal and more as a result of breaking down the higher fat, higher energy ingredients that are in most wet foods.

Less stress. The "body-mind connection" works for cats just as well as it does for people. Country folks know that a healthy attitude toward life makes for a healthy body. Unfortunately, you can't explain that to your cat. Instead, it's up to you to minimize his stress and maximize his health.

Try to anticipate problems. Do you know a major change is coming up in your household? Whether it's a new baby, someone going off to college for the first time, a family vacation, or remodeling the kitchen, if you know it's coming it's best to either ease the cat into it slowly or expect an attack of urinary problems and take the necessary precautions. (An example of the easing-in-slowly strategy is a new baby: Set up the nursery ahead of time; if you're going to keep the cat out of that room, start doing it before the baby is born; or bring in a supply of whatever lotions, creams, or wipes you're going to have so the cat has time to get used to the new smells.)

You should have realistic expectations for your cat. Sure, cats are clever and agile and maybe even a little sneaky, but they're still cats. It's entirely possible that your cat understands everything you say and is just playing dumb or being obstinate. However, it's equally possible that he's only learned how to get along in human society just well enough to find himself a comfortable situation and doesn't have a clue why you're so bent out of shape that he's been urinating in your beautiful potted plants instead of the convenient litter box you bought him.

Chapter 7, "Behavior and Training" goes into more detail on the best ways to shape your cat's behavior to make you both happy. For now, let's just say that those stories you hear about cats peeing in their owner's shoes to "get even" may not be far from the truth. If a cat doesn't understand why he's being reprimanded, he stresses out. A stressed cat will announce his unhappiness with a change in behavior, often by elimination. And, to a cat, leaving it where you're sure to notice it—where your personal smell is strongest—is a great way to guarantee you'll get the message.

Finally, to lessen your cat's stress, try to stay cool yourself. Have you ever tried to enjoy a favorite activity and then had someone who was really, really intense about it right next to you? To cats, life in your home is basically one long stay at a resort hotel: The weather is always fine, everything is already paid for, you don't have to work, and you can eat, sleep, and play whenever you feel like it. If the humans in this little paradise are under stress, though, the vacation is suddenly over. Some of this may be cats' fabled sensitivity to people's emotions, but some of it certainly is a reaction to the changes in the way we humans move and speak when we're agitated.

Check the box. A clean litter box filled with the appropriate kind of litter must be available to the cat at all times. Using the litter box is not an instinctive behavior in cats; the instinct part is the action of

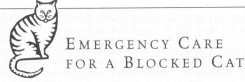

EMERGENCY CARE FOR A BLOCKED CAT

What if your cat blocks up in the middle of the night, while you're away at work, or without any warning signs? Several hours can pass before the blockage can be noticed, and by that time, the cat may be in serious trouble. It's a life-or-death situation, and you may have to try and unblock the cat yourself.

First, be aware of three important points:

• Every second counts, so its best to try unblocking the cat while you're in the process of getting him to the vet

• While urinary blockage is extremely painful, unblocking usually hurts even more; even the nicest cat will bite or scratch when in pain

• Even if you're successful in unblocking the cat, he still needs prompt veterinary care.

digging in loose materials to bury their urine and feces (especially if there is a habit of using that spot or the very faint residual smell of elimination there). If something turns them off to the box (like it's too dirty, too perfumey, or too much trouble to get to), they'll either hold it too long (increasing bladder irritation and the risk of infection) or find another "toilet." (See the section on litter box accidents in Chapter 8, "Common Behavorial Problems and Home Remedies.") Check your cat's litter box regularly, making sure it is clean and free of irritants.

To unblock a cat, it's best to have the assistance of another person. Have the other person use one hand to apply pressure over the cat's shoulders, forcing the cat firmly down while using the other hand to hold one or both of the cat's back legs. Now lift the cat's tail to expose its hind end. Grasp the urinary opening between your thumb and forefinger, and gently wiggle back and forth. You can also use a "milking" motion, going from the body outward. Either of these may produce mucous or a white, gritty-looking substance, possibly tinged with blood. If the obstruction breaks loose, urine usually starts to flow.

Occasionally, a blockage can be pushed loose by gently squeezing the bladder. Put your hand around the cat's underbelly, just in front of the back legs. Squeeze with even pressure but not too hard or too long—since the bladder can't empty, it's stretched tight and can rupture.

☎ WHEN TO CALL THE VET

Cats with urinary tract problems will often deliberately urinate outside of the litter box, even if they've been 100 percent accurate all their lives. If your cat suddenly starts having "accidents," spraying urine, or squatting and straining outside of the box, don't punish him. He's probably telling you he's got a problem. Call the vet as soon as you notice one of these signals and schedule an appointment for an exam. If it's a physical problem, the sooner your catch it, the

Common Physical Problems and Home Remedies

easier it will be to treat. If it's a purely behavioral thing, you can start correcting it before it becomes an ingrained habit.

If your cat is straining in the litter box (or elsewhere) and not producing any urine, produces small amounts of bloody urine, or cries during urination, call the vet immediately. These are the signs of a urinary blockage, an extremely serious—and potentially fatal—problem. (See the section on urinary blockage in Chapter 4, "What Every Cat Owner Should Know.")

✳ DANGER LEVEL: Most bladder problems by themselves are not dangerous; they're mostly inconvenient and a nuisance for the owner. However, urinary blockage is extremely dangerous and should be treated as a life-threatening situation.

DANDRUFF / ITCHY SKIN

WHAT IT IS

Those same little white flakes that sell millions of dollars of medicated shampoo to human consumers can afflict cats as well. Since a cat has hair all over her body, dandruff is easy to spot. The flakes are dead, dried-out skin and usually the result of some sort of allergic dermatitis—a reaction to something that makes the cat's skin dry, itchy, or scaly.

The causes of allergic dermatitis can be anything from parasites—such as fleas or mites—to sunburn, to a sensitivity to new carpeting, or even to something as simple as the air being too dry during heating season. Don't confuse dandruff—the result of abnormally dry or itchy skin—with dander. Dander refers to normal shedding of dead skin cells, combined with proteins in the cat's saliva, left on the hair and skin when the cat grooms herself. (This dander isn't the result of an allergic reaction in the cat, but it is the cause of allergies to cats in humans.)

Homeopathy for Cats

Homeopathic medicine is one of the more popular "alternative" healing methods. Actually, its basic principle dates back some 3,000 years and was later expounded by Hippocrates. "Modern" homeopathy dates back almost 200 years to a time when blood-letting was the major form of mainstream medical treatment.

Homeopathy is based on the idea that like cures like. The classic example is quinine: It cures malaria; but given to a healthy person, it produces the symptoms of malaria. However, homeopathic remedies are not simply preparations of the plant or mineral products after which they're named. The remedies are prepared by a careful series of dilutions and succussion (vigorous shaking) until little, if any, of the original material is left. These dilutions are called potencies, and the more dilutions and succussion done, the higher the potency of the remedy. Homeopathy is also a truly holistic discipline. A homeopathic physician (or veterinarian) looks for the single remedy that best fits the overall condition of the patient, not just the most recent severe symptoms.

Homeopathy for animals isn't a new idea, either; homeopaths have been treating dogs, cats, and farm animals for at least the last 50 years. Today there are a number of vets specifically trained in homeopathy. Contact the National Center for Homeopathy (see Chapter 9, "Where to Learn More") for more information.

What's the humidity? If you feel like the air is dry in your home and your skin feels dry and tight as a result, you can bet your cat is experiencing the same thing. Humidifying will not only lick the dry skin problem, it will cut down on static electricity in your cat's coat and reduce the likelihood of winter colds.

Look for freeloaders. Check your cat for parasites. Bites from fleas, lice, and mites can all cause allergic dermatitis. Chyletiella mites have been called "walking dandruff" since they're large enough to see with the naked eye but too small to distinguish detail. All skin parasites can be treated fairly easily, but in order to stamp them out completely, you'll probably have to treat all other animals in the home, the house itself, and sometimes even the people.

Made in the shade. A cat's coat protects the sensitive skin underneath from the burning rays of the sun. But cats that spend a lot of time outdoors can still get sunburn, especially on the tips of their ears, eyelids, nose, or lips. Any place the hair is sparse—the area on the head above the eye and below the ear or wherever the cat has scars or bald patches—are particularly sensitive. Sunburn kills the top layer of skin, which dries up and flakes off. Repeated sunburn can cause skin cancer—another reason to keep cats indoors. At the very least, cats that have had a sunburn or are especially at risk for it (cats with thin, sparse, or white coats, for example) should be kept indoors during the most intense period of ultraviolet (burning) sun rays—generally from about 10:00 o'clock in the morning to 3:00 or 4:00 o'clock in the afternoon.

☎ WHEN TO CALL THE VET

Persistent or worsening itching and flaking or the presence of parasites calls for professional veterinary care. Over-the-counter pet shampoos and parasite treatments usually aren't potent enough to do the trick.

DANGER LEVEL: Most causes of dandruff are not dangerous. But, if left untreated, some causes may be so uncomfortable that the cat scratches herself raw, running a mildly dangerous risk of infection.

DEAFNESS/BLINDNESS

WHAT IT IS

Cats can lose hearing or vision in accidents, as a result of disease, or because of birth defects. Reactions to some medications or lack of oxygen during birth can also impair hearing and sight.

If a cat doesn't get enough of the amino acid taurine in her diet, her retinas (the layer of light-sensitive cells inside the eyeball that send messages about sight to the brain) can deteriorate, causing blindness. All-white cats with blue eyes have a high risk of being deaf, a condition related to Waardenburg syndrome in humans. White cats with yellow eyes or one blue eye have a greater than normal chance of being deaf, although not as likely as blue-eyed white cats.

WHAT TO DO ABOUT IT

Find the reason. When vision starts going bad because of diet, switching to the right kind of food can often stop—but not reverse—the deterioration. On the other hand, cataracts (cloudy lenses in the eyes) can be corrected surgically, just like in people. A thorough veterinary exam can determine if a cat's hearing loss is treatable (for example, an obstruction in the ear canal like impacted wax, ear mite debris, or a tumor) or not.

Make adjustments. Incredibly, blind cats can eventually figure out the layout of their home, more or less by the Braille method. You may want to keep a blind cat restricted to certain rooms or levels of the house to avoid accidental tumbles down stairs or exits out external doors. Once a blind cat learns the lay of the land at home, do your utmost not to change anything. If a door is usually open, leave it open. If furniture has to be moved for some reason, put it back where it was. A blind cat relies on landmarks that are at cat level—just a few inches off the floor—so even something as simple as leaving shoes in the hallway can throw her off.

Seeing (and feeling) is believing. Deaf cats process the world through their sense of sight and touch. The feline eye perceives moving objects better than stationary ones, so deaf cats take particular pleasure in making things move—especially downward from high places to shatter below. The thuds, crashes, and smashes that would send a hearing cat running for cover are lost on a deaf cat. Any visually stimulating thing is particularly interesting to deaf cats, so their owners should take note and try to provide them—or to prevent them, if they're unsafe or unwelcome. For example, owners should remove breakable knick-knacks from shelves so ambitious cats can't knock them off.

> Kittens usually open their eyes nine days after birth. The exception is Siamese, whose eyes tend to open earlier.

Sound is felt as vibrations in the deaf world. You may not be able to get your cat's attention by calling her name, or you may not be able to reprimand her with a sharp "No!" However, you can do both by stamping your foot or knocking on whatever surface the cat happens to occupy.

The golden years. All the senses and body functions slow down with advancing age, and hearing and vision are no exceptions. Once a cat passes middle age (anywhere from six to ten years old), expect her to lose a little of her edge. The difference with an elderly cat whose vision or hearing has gone down is that her other faculties have diminished, too, and she can't adapt as well. She also has a lifetime habit of relying on full-functioning eyes and ears. At that point, the

Common Physical Problems and Home Remedies

most important ingredient for dealing with a blind or deaf cat is patience—she's doing the best she can with what she has.

☎ WHEN TO CALL THE VET

If your cat seems to be less responsive to sound, bumps into things, or her pupils stay dilated even in bright light, contact your vet for an evaluation.

✳ DANGER LEVEL: Deafness and blindness themselves are not dangerous. However, deaf and blind cats are at a serious disadvantage once they leave the familiarity of their own home. It's not only extremely dangerous to let a deaf or blind cat outdoors unattended, it's cruel.

DIABETES

WHAT IT IS

The pancreas is a long gland that lies directly beneath the stomach. A cluster of specialized cells in the pancreas produce insulin, which regulates the body's uptake and breakdown of sugar. Diabetes mellitus (usually just called diabetes or sugar diabetes) is the result of a shortage of insulin. Diabetics have intense thirst, produce large amounts of urine, and have abnormally high levels of sugar in their blood and urine. Other signs of diabetes are increased appetite and slow healing.

Left untreated, the diabetic cat will lose weight (despite eating more) and become lethargic. Later signs of untreated diabetes include vomiting, diarrhea, rapid breathing, weakness, and finally collapse and death.

Your vet's diagnosis of diabetes is based on the cat's clinical signs, physical exam findings, and laboratory test results, primarily a persistent presence of abnormally high levels of sugar in the blood and urine.

Diabetes is a disease of older cats, rarely occurring before the age of seven years. It can be managed through diet and, when necessary, supplementary insulin. With treatment, diabetic cats can live ordinary lives, and a few may return to normal function for reasons that are not well understood.

What to do about it

Watch that weight. Obese cats are more likely to develop diabetes. In fact, cats who weigh in at 15 pounds or more have double the risk of diabetes than the under-15-pound crowd. Keeping your cat's weight under control is a simple formula: Feed only the recommended amounts, limit (or eliminate) snacks and treats, and make sure Tabby stays active.

You are what you eat. A high-fiber diet helps control diabetes by regulating the rate at which nutrients are taken into body cells. This, in turn, keeps blood sugar levels more consistent. Feeding several small meals during the day has a similar effect on blood sugar. A couple of large meals spread several hours apart cause a post-meal blood sugar surge, followed by a below-normal level by the time the next meal comes around. A normal cat's body smooths out these peaks and valleys, but it's a problem for diabetics. Many diabetic cats can have their blood sugar levels returned to normal through diet and weight loss alone.

Himmy, a tabby cat from Australia, weighed just under 47 pounds when he died. He was the world's largest cat.

Be prepared. One of the most important aspects of managing the health of a diabetic cat is consistency. Food and medication must come at regular times, so be sure you always have an adequate supply of both and never skip or substitute.

Occasionally, a diabetic cat on insulin will have her blood sugar level suddenly swing dangerously to the low side—a condition known as hypoglycemia. Signs of hypoglycemia include shaking, disorientation, salivating, staggering and falling, and seizures. Keep an emergency sugar source on hand at all times (honey or Karo syrup are the usual recommendations). At the first sign of hypoglycemia, rub some on the cat's gums—and call the vet immediately.

☎ When to call the vet

If your cat shows signs of diabetes, schedule a veterinary exam as soon as possible. The longer a diabetic cat goes untreated, the more serious her condition gets. The earlier you can catch and control her diabetes, the more likely she is to have a normal lifespan.

A cat who's already being treated for diabetes needs to go to the vet immediately if she shows signs of hypoglycemia or any kind of reaction to her medication.

✳ DANGER LEVEL: Untreated diabetes and hypoglycemia are extremely dangerous; however, both can be treated and controlled.

Diarrhea

What it is

When the body needs to get rid of something quickly, it speeds up the action of the intestines and cuts down on water reabsorbtion from the gut. The end result (no pun intended) of this important defense mechanism is diarrhea. Once the cat's body has expelled the suspect stuff—and no more is taken in—diarrhea usually clears up by itself.

Certain viruses and diseases, a change in diet, or a food allergy can also trigger diarrhea. In the case of illness or food allergy, the diarrhea may not clear up for several days. Because it also removes fluid from the body, bouts lasting more than 24 hours may cause dehydration (see the section on hydration in Chapter 5, "At-Home Health Care: Practical Skills"), which is a potentially serious condition.

An occasional loose stool or bout of diarrhea is a normal part of life and will pass without you having to do anything. When a cat suffers "the runs" for more than a day, though, you may need to help nature along.

What's the cause? Make a mental checklist of the previous 24 hours. Did your cat rummage through the garbage? Have a snack of "people" food? Eat a new food of any kind? Have a major stress or trauma (such as a plane trip)? Now think about the past week. Has there been an increase in stress for the cat? Did she eat some nonfood item? Has she been showing other symptoms of illness? These are all questions to ask yourself when evaluating your cat's condition.

Try the "quiet diet." The less work your cat's digestive system has to do, the faster it will settle back into its normal functioning.

You'll need to keep dairy products away from your cat. Although cats love dairy products, they don't digest them well. A saucer of milk or cream may be the storybook feline snack, but the lactose (milk sugar) in dairy products frequently is a cause of diarrhea.

Get rid of cat foods that contain dyes. Cat food that comes in attractive colors, is processed to look like chunks of meat, or stays moist in the container for months include dyes and other artificial ingredients. These are nonfoods, and the gut has to work harder to process them—just the opposite of what you want for a cat with diarrhea. Although changing foods also can cause diarrhea, switching over to a brand with no dyes or additives can help clear up the current trouble and prevent future bouts.

Try to give your cat foods that are easy on the stomach. Cooked white rice mixed with boiled hamburger or chicken meat is bland and easy to digest. Some cats balk at rice, so you may have to use potatoes or pasta instead. If you don't feel like cooking for your cat, lamb and rice cat foods are available at most pet supply stores.

You can also try fasting your cat. Sometimes fasting your cat for 24 hours is enough to drop the intestines back into low gear. If nothing at all goes in (except water), there's nothing to process; and by the end of the 24 hours, nothing should be coming out. When you resume feeding, begin with the bland rice mixture, then slowly mix in regular food, reducing the amount of the rice mixture until the cat is back on a normal diet.

If Not Nature . . . Although common sense says that adding a stool-softening laxative to your cat's food will keep the bowels moving, a bulk-forming laxative such as Metamucil seems to have a normalizing effect on cats with diarrhea. If your cat's stools are still a little soft during or after a couple of days of the "quiet diet," try adding about a half-teaspoon of the Metamucil laxative to each of her meals for a day or two.

Keep her hydrated. It's important that a cat with diarrhea keeps drinking. In fact, her need for fluids is actually greater, so make sure she has plenty of water available at all times. Besides losing fluids, though, a cat with diarrhea is losing key nutrients called electrolytes. These nutrients, such as sodium and potassium, make the nerves work right. To replenish electrolytes, keep fluid intake at the necessary level and provide some extra energy boost; you can try filling a bowl with Gatorade sports drink.

Nature's way. Nature provides its own way to slow down and get back to normal. Relaxation, stress reduction, and gentle exercise (take your cat for a walk on a leash and harness, if she likes it) may be all that are needed to clear up a attack of loose stools. Avoid the temptation to use over-the-counter diarrhea products, unless your vet specifically tells you to.

Call the vet immediately if severe (watery or "explosive") diarrhea continues for more than 24 hours or if diarrhea worsens, is bloody, or is accompanied by other symptoms such as vomiting, fever, or difficulty walking. A cat with diarrhea should drink a little more, but intense thirst with diarrhea may be a sign of diabetes.

✳ DANGER LEVEL: By itself, diarrhea is only slightly dangerous, mostly because of the risks of dehydration. Severe, bloody, or watery diarrhea—or diarrhea accompanied by other symptoms of illness—can be a sign of something as routine as worms or as serious as panleukopenia (feline distemper).

EAR MITES

WHAT THEY ARE

Tiny, pinpoint-size ear mites live and breed in the ear canals of cats and dogs. They feed on skin debris and can gnaw on the tissue of the ear canal, using cell fluids and blood for food, too. Ear mite infestations usually itch, so cats with ear mites will scratch excessively at the backs or insides of their ears (sometimes to the point of producing raw patches), shake their heads, or hold their ears at an angle to their heads.

Ear mites produce a black or brownish waxy debris in the ear canal, which looks very much like coffee grounds. Live mites can be seen in this debris with a hand lens or by spreading a small amount on dark paper and watching for tiny, moving white points.

Treatment of ear mites involves removing the debris from the ears and using a topical insecticide in the canal for a period of time to kill off the remaining mites and new mites that hatch out of eggs left behind. Since the mites can crawl out of the ear canal and onto the cat's fur—or the fur of other animals—all animals in the house should be dusted, sprayed, or dipped with an antiflea product. Ear mites are extremely common, and treatment is usually inexpensive and effective.

WHAT TO DO ABOUT IT

If your cat has itchy ears and you see the telltale debris in the ear canal, gently remove a little bit of the junk with a cotton ball and examine it under bright light with a hand lens or spread it on a piece of dark paper. Any movement—including tiny white moving specks—means mites. Sometimes, mite debris is located deep in the ear canal where you can't see it. If you suspect your cat has mites, gently massage the back of the ear at the base between your thumb and forefinger. A cat with no mites usually enjoys it or, at worst, will fuss and try to get away. A cat who has unwanted company living in her ear canal will usually start scratching vigorously so watch your hand because she won't.

Other ear problems can cause itchiness and debris in the ear canal, too, so don't start home remedies for ear mites until you're fairly certain that's the problem. Seeing live mites is real proof. When you have that proof, try to ease your cat's discomfort.

Clean them out. The first step toward clearing up an ear mite infestation is to get as many tiny critters (and their belongings) out of the ear canal as possible. Put several drops of mineral oil into the ear canal and massage gently. If the debris is particularly hard and crusty, you may have to let the oil work in for a few hours to soften things up. The massaging will help bring debris up to the outer part of the ear where it can be wiped away with a cotton ball or tissue. (Do not use cotton swabs, even though you may have seen your vet clean your cat's ears that way—one slip could puncture an eardrum.) If you want to do a thorough cleaning job (and you're courageous enough), you can use lukewarm distilled water in an ear syringe to gently flush out the canal. Repeat the cleaning procedure until the debris is gone.

Hit them while they're down. While the mineral oil immobilizes any mites left behind, it won't kill them all. To do that, you need insecticide ear drops. Reliable products that contain pyrethrins (a natural insecticide found in flowers of the mum family) are widely available at pet supply stores. Follow directions carefully, making sure to massage the drops in well and wipe away any excess.

Where mites might be. By the time you notice your cat has ear mites, there are literally thousands of the itty-bitty things around. Smaller than the period at the end of this sentence, a single ear mite can crawl out of your cat's ear canal and hide out deep in her fur— only to crawl back in after all the excitement of treatment is over and repopulate the colony. Therefore, cats with ear mites need regular treatment with flea products to knock out those adventurous mites that go exploring elsewhere on the cat's body.

Once is not enough. A single cleaning and treatment with ear drops won't do the trick. Just one surviving female mite with eggs can have your cat right back where you started from before you know it. You must be absolutely diligent about cleaning out your cat's ears every day or two and using the medication exactly as directed. It's not enough to kill all the mites in your cat's ears, either. Microscopic mite eggs can hatch days after a treatment, starting the infestation all over again. It usually takes a few weeks of treatment before you can safely assume your cat and home are ear-mite-free.

☎ WHEN TO CALL THE VET

If your best home remedies don't knock out ear mites within a month or the skin in or around the ear becomes raw or inflamed, you need professional help. Likewise, if your cat has itchy ears, shakes her head, flattens her ears, and has discharge from the ear canal—but no mite debris or there are no live mites to be found—check with your vet. It could be a yeast or bacterial infection or another type of ear problem.

✳ DANGER LEVEL: Ear mites are annoying and sometimes painful to the cat but not dangerous. They're contagious to dogs and other cats, and untreated infestations may lead to excessive scratching and wounds behind the ears that may become infected.

FELINE IMMUNODEFICIENY VIRUS (FIV), FELINE INFECTIOUS PERITONITIS (FIP), AND FELINE LEUKEMIA VIRUS (FELV)

WHAT THEY ARE

FIV, FIP, and FeLV are three extremely serious, incurable, and usually fatal cat diseases caused by viruses. Each is caused by a different kind of virus. However, they are all contagious only between cats, are nearly 100 percent fatal once they cause serious illness, and have the interesting quirk that not all cats exposed to them will get sick.

Unlike the viruses that cause upper respiratory diseases or distemper in cats and can be carried in the air, these three require the physical presence of an infected cat in the same place (although not necessarily at the same time) as the cat who catches it. FIP and FeLV are spread most often by pro-longed close contact with an infected cat. Close contact can include

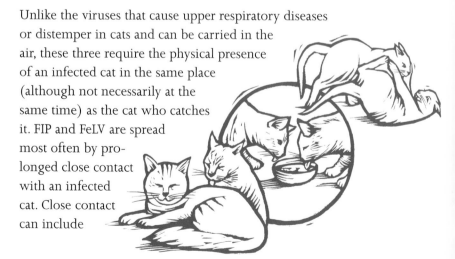

mutual grooming or sharing food, water, elimination areas, or sleeping quarters. This means a cat who goes outdoors and urinates or defecates where a cat carrying FIP or FeLV goes can catch the virus without ever having had physical contact with the carrier. FIP and FeLV can also be spread to kittens by a mother with the virus.

The main route of infection for FIV appears to be a bite from an infected cat. Cats who go outdoors—particularly if they fight—are therefore at risk. The most common profile of an FIV-positive cat is an unneutered male who goes outdoors and has sustained bites and scratches from other cats.

Cats who appear otherwise healthy may be carrying these viruses. Reliable blood tests exist for FeLV and FIV. There is a test for FIP; however, a positive FIP test alone—without other symptoms or risk factors—is not absolute proof the cat has the virus.

FIV is sometimes also called feline AIDS (or FAIDS). FIV does have a few general similarities to HIV, the virus associated with AIDS: It belongs to the same class of viruses, can stay in the body for years without causing illness, and when it becomes active, slowly breaks down the disease-fighting immune system. However, AIDS is a human disease, and FIV cannot infect humans.

What to do about them

There's no question that these three diseases are scary. Once any one of them starts making your cat sick, there's not much that can be done other than to make the cat as comfortable as possible for as long as she has to live. The good news is these diseases can be prevented and, in many cases, with 100 percent success.

Take the test. Since a cat can appear healthy and still carry one of these viruses, a new arrival—even your first cat—should be tested for FeLV. Kittens probably don't need FIV tests unless they were strays, but it's probably a good idea to test adult cats from any source. Your veterinarian may recommend a retest in a few months. This isn't a scam; if your cat was very recently infected, it may not show up on the first test.

Stop the spread. There's only one surefire way to prevent your cat from contracting FeLV, FIP, or FIV: Keep her away from the sources of the viruses. In other words, keep her away from other cats and the places they frequent. This usually means keeping cats indoors at all times. It definitely means testing any new cat added to your household for FeLV and FIV before she's allowed to meet the resident cat or have run of any of the same areas. Preventative vaccines are available for FeLV and FIP. Schedule an appointment with your vet to talk about the advisability of vaccinating your cats for these diseases.

Be positive about positives. If your cat tests positive for FeLV or FIV and a retest confirms it, don't give up hope. With good care, FeLV- and FIV-positive cats can live for years, even after signs of disease appear. New treatments are coming all the time, and there may be a breakthrough that will help your cat long before she gets seriously ill. Be responsible about the news. Keep your cat away from uninfected cats, and don't add any FeLV- or FIV-negative cats to your household. It may be tempting to start taking in other FeLV- and FIV-positive cats who are facing euthanasia, but think it over carefully. Eventually, the disease will catch up with them, and they'll demand a lot of time and resources. It may be best to focus on the special status of your own cat and give her the best possible quality of life.

Treat the symptoms. Most of what you can do for cats who are sick with FeLV, FIP, or FIV is just make them feel better. This might be as simple as indulging them with their favorite foods when their appetites are poor or coaxing them to eat with petting and hand-feeding. However, each virus has its signature complications that may also need attention, usually from the vet and with follow-up or nursing care at home. FeLV causes lymphosarcoma, a kind of cancerous tumor that may need to be removed. The "wet" (effusive) form of FIP causes fluid to build up in the chest, making breathing difficult, or in the abdomen, giving the cat a bloated appearance. This buildup is a problem your vet can sometimes relieve by suctioning out the fluid with a needle and syringe. Since FIV attacks the immune system, you'll have to stay on top of secondary infections with prevention and medication.

☎ WHEN TO CALL THE VET

These three viral diseases are a strong case for annual veterinary checkups. The early signs of any of the diseases are often too subtle for the average cat owner to notice, but a veterinarian knows what to look for. In between checkups, notify your vet of any sudden abdominal bloating or swelling, low-grade signs of illness that never quite go away (sneezing or diarrhea, for example), any lumps on your cat's body, or bites or scratches from cats not known to be FeLV- and FIV-negative.

Cats who have been diagnosed with FeLV, FIP, or FIV should see the vet regularly.

☀ DANGER LEVEL: All three of these diseases (FeLV, FIP, and FIV) are extremely dangerous. Although surprisingly few cats exposed to these viruses will get sick from them, once the illness begins it is almost always fatal.

FLEAS

WHAT THEY ARE

These small, flat-bodied insects are no bigger than a pinhead, yet they have literally conquered the world. Fleas are found just about everywhere, they are tough to kill, and they can leap many times their body length.

Fleas can live off the blood of just about any warm-blooded animal, but they prefer the higher body temperature of dogs and cats over humans. They reproduce quickly, and their eggs can survive in the environment for long periods of time—time enough to hatch out and take over the skin of the next host that happens by.

In areas that have cold winters, outdoor fleas die off (although untreated indoor infestations can last year-round). In warm and humid regions like south Florida and Louisiana, however, "flea season" is a year-round event.

A cat with fleas may scratch a lot, but then again, she may not. Surefire signs of fleas are small, black comma-shaped droppings in the cat's coat and, of course, the presence of live fleas. Both may be noticeable when the cat is being combed or brushed—another good reason for regular grooming. To check a cat for flea dirt, stand her on a white or light-colored surface and ruffle her fur vigorously. If you see black specks around her, moisten a cotton ball or tissue and smear the specks. A streak of blood confirms flea dirt.

> Fleas in Florida are now resistant to nearly all of the most common flea treatments.

What to do about it

Make no mistake about it, when your cat has fleas, you are going to war against an enemy that is not about to surrender. You have to wipe it out or put it into retreat down to the last man, woman, and child. There's no such thing as peaceful coexistence.

Kill them on the cat. Forget over-the-counter flea sprays and powders—they're just not strong enough. You need a professional-strength flea treatment, which means going to your vet or a groomer. Flea collars are also very little help in the battle against fleas. A plastic band with time-released insecticide at your cat's neck isn't going to do much to kill fleas riding on your cat's tail. Worse, if flea collars get wet, some can release all of their poison at once.

Kill them in your home. If your cat has fleas, your house has fleas. Not a pleasant thought, but true. If you just bathe, dip, or spray the cat, any fleas not killed will immediately abandon ship (remember their astounding jumping ability) and wait until the coast is clear to return to your cat. Or, they may switch over to a human host for awhile until the pesticide on your cat is gone. Actually, treating the cat for fleas is the easy part (although it may not seem like it at the time). Treating your home is more complicated.

"Evict" fleas from your home by thoroughly vacuuming the entire house, including floors, carpets, and upholstery. Immediately dispose of the vacuum cleaner bag in an outdoor garbage can. In hot water, wash the bedding and linen from anywhere the cat sleeps.

The next step is to "bomb" the annoying insects. Cover or securely put away all dishes, eating utensils, baby or pet toys, and other items. Remove all pets and people from the home, and set off the appropriate number of insecticide foggers for the size and number of rooms of your house. Use veterinary-strength foggers, not over-the-counter house or yard products. A good way to coordinate tactics is to take the infested animals for their flea baths or dips while the foggers are doing their work. You'll probably have to stay out of the house for a few hours after the foggers have been set off.

Even if you've been successful in killing every flea on your pets and in your home, there can still be flea eggs left behind. You'll probably have to repeat the treatments again to catch these stragglers as they hatch out. Newer flea products contain growth regulators that prevent eggs and young fleas from maturing, which can make things easier; however, some people may be allergic to these chemicals.

Common Physical Problems and Home Remedies

Keep them out. You may have defeated the enemy on the home front, but you've only won the battle—the war goes on. Cats who go outdoors are almost guaranteed to pick up fleas again. Fleas can also be brought back inside to indoor cats by the family dog. Even without a dog to serve as the "flea train," though, the more the door and unscreened windows are open during flea season, the more likely one or more of those hardy little critters are to hop into your home. Regular preventative flea treatment in your home will help prevent a sneak attack.

☎ WHEN TO CALL THE VET

As soon as you see live fleas or flea dirt on your cat, call your vet. The longer you wait, the more fleas you'll have to fight. Your vet can give you the shampoos, foams, dips, sprays, topical treatments, oral medications, and foggers you'll need for your war on fleas, or you can have the vet or groomer do the treatment on the animals.

✳ DANGER LEVEL: Fleas are mostly a nuisance and only slightly dangerous. They can carry tapeworms, which your cat can only get by swallowing a flea. A cat who has a particularly bad case of fleas can lose so much blood she becomes anemic. Anemia is moderately to very dangerous for kittens and weakened cats.

HAIR LOSS (ALOPECIA)

WHAT IT IS

Cats shed constantly, so there's a certain amount of natural hair loss every cat owner should expect. However, bald patches, "hot spots" (areas that are inflamed and red and that the cat may lick or scratch excessively), and hair that gets so sparse you can see the skin underneath are all signs of a problem.

Hair loss happens for reasons as simple as a scar to more serious causes such as skin fungus, mites or fleas, or hormonal imbalances.

Dermatitis is another word for inflamed skin, and many kinds of dermatitis result in hair loss, too. Stress can also cause hair loss. A stressed cat not only sheds more but a very anxious cat may actually tear out her own hair by excessive licking or chewing.

What to do about it

Location, location, location. If the hair loss is someplace you see your cat licking, biting, or scratching regularly (leg, paw, or side, for example), it could be a "hot spot" that is stress-induced or a reaction to bites from fleas or mites. Check your cat's coat for parasites. If it's a flea-bite allergy, you'll have to get rid of the fleas before you can hope to have the hair grow back. If the hair loss is in a hard-to-reach place (between the shoulder blades, for example) or in many places, it's probably not the cat doing it to herself. If the hair loss seems limited to one area of the body (for example, on the legs from the paws up to the "elbows"), suspect a "contact allergy" or something similar. (Hair loss on the lower legs may be a reaction to new carpeting.)

You are what you eat. Have you been cutting corners on food costs by giving Tabby an off-brand or trying to go with table scraps only? Hair loss can be a sign of improper nutrition, so make sure your cat is getting the nutrients she needs.

Less stress is best. Actually, this advice could be added to every remedy! However, once your cat develops the habit of chewing, licking, or pulling out hair, it might be hard to break even after you cut down on stress. Do not scold or otherwise punish your cat when you see her working on a "hot spot" or pulling out hair. Scolding just adds more stress. Instead, try some behavior modification. Give her something else to do: Engage her in active play, pet her, open a securely screened window and let her sniff the great outdoors. Substituting a happy and fun activity for the bad habit redirects her attention and energy.

Common Physical Problems and Home Remedies

A cat with hair loss plus other signs of disease—fever, loss of appetite, weight loss, vomiting—needs to be seen by a veterinarian immediately. Certain kinds of alopecia are caused by parasites or fungus that can be passed to people, so the sooner a cat with no other symptoms than hair loss is seen by the vet, the better.

✳ DANGER LEVEL: Alopecia by itself is not dangerous, although it may be a signal that internal organs are not working right—a condition that could be moderately to very dangerous.

HAIRBALLS

WHAT THEY ARE

Every time your cat grooms herself, she swallows some loose hairs. The hairs don't digest and then they get passed through the cat's stomach and intestines. Sometimes—especially in longhair cats, during periods of heavy shedding, or in cats who groom other cats or groom themselves excessively—the cat swallows enough hair so that it forms a wad in the cat's stomach. These wads of hair are ejected as hairballs.

Virtually all cats have hairballs at some point in their lives. Many are passed through the intestines, but cats who swallow large amounts of fur can develop hairballs that actually clog the digestive system and have to be removed with surgery.

WHAT TO DO ABOUT IT

Many times, the best thing to do when your cat coughs up a hairball is...nothing (except clean it up, of course). Once the hairball is out, everything's usually fine. Still, if your cat is bringing up hairballs regularly or to prevent future hairballs, there are some tried-and-true tricks to take care of this common cat complaint.

TALES FROM THE COUNTRY VET: ALTERNATIVE MEDICINE FOR CATS

"You should try acupuncture for your bad back," someone once told my old pal, Hoke Mitchell. "The Chinese have been using it for thousands of years." "Yeah," quipped Hoke, "but are any of them alive today?"

The truth is, there's a lot more interest in these sorts of things now than in living memory. I think that's good. As long as it doesn't hurt the cat, might make her feel better, and doesn't blind you to the obvious (giving herbs to a cat with a broken leg is great, but she also needs a splint and cast).

Acupuncture is, of course, the use of tiny needles placed in strategic locations to help healing energy flow in the body. There are plenty of studies that show its success on people, and there's no reason to believe animals can't benefit, too. Those who are squeamish about needles can try acupressure, which involves pressing on the points instead of sticking them. Naturopathy is a whole system of helping get the body back to full health by restoring natural balance. Some alternative methods, such as homeopathy and chiropractic, are already used regularly and widely for humans. Other choices include herbs, flower essences, and gemstones.

If you're interested in alternative medicine for your cat, find a vet who is knowledgeable in this area. Chapter 9, "Where to Learn More," will help you find one.

Common Physical Problems and Home Remedies

Brush up a bit. Regular grooming, even just a little bit every few days, removes the loose hairs that cause hairballs. Remember, every loose hair you brush or comb off your cat is one less for her to swallow.

Ease the passing. A small amount of intestinal lubrication will help hairballs make their way through the digestive system instead of coming back up. You can buy commercial hairball remedies, use a little bit of melted butter, or give your cat a small dollop of petroleum jelly. The petroleum jelly is probably the cheapest and most effective method, but it's also the one most difficult to convince the cat to swallow. Butter is probably a better bet, since most cats love dairy and fat. Give your cat about a half-teaspoon of melted butter once a day for a few days (and no longer); it should do the trick. Commercial remedies taste good and are very effective, but always read and follow label directions carefully. (Never give any hairball remedy as a daily part of the cat's diet or for more than four or five days in a row, unless specifically recommended by your veterinarian.)

Bulk up your cat's diet. Too many snacks, too little fiber, and not enough exercise. It may sound like what the doctor told you at your last checkup, but it's equally sound advice for your cat. A hairball is a problem because it just sits there. Unless you get your cat's system moving a little more vigorously, hair will continue to collect, form hairballs, and be thrown up on your best rug or next to the bed for you to find with your bare feet in the middle of the night. A higher fiber diet, fewer empty-calorie snacks, and a little more exercise may be all it takes to lick a hairball problem.

A hairball once in awhile is normal. Hairballs several times a week or even daily is a problem. Hairballs usually come up in one or two tries. If your cat continues retching and trying to bring something up or has diarrhea that won't stop or loses her appetite along with hairballs, call your vet right away. It doesn't happen often, but hairballs can get so bad they block the throat, stomach, or intestines; and that can be fatal.

☀ DANGER LEVEL: Occasional hairballs should be considered normal, and even more frequent ones are not dangerous. If hairballs can't be passed or thrown up, though, they can cause blockages in the digestive system that are very dangerous.

KIDNEY FAILURE

WHAT IT IS

The kidneys' major job is filtering out wastes. Age, injury, or disease can damage and destroy the function of kidney tissue. The body can adjust to minor kidney damage or the early stages of kidney failure, so there may be no noticeable signs at first. As damage or failure worsens, a cat produces more urine and drinks more to compensate. In the later stages of failure, the kidneys can't keep up the pace, and wastes back up in the body, poisoning the cat and causing vomiting, loss of appetite, weight loss, and often telltale "ammonia breath."

Unfortunately, once kidney failure reaches this point, it's usually irreversible. The best way to detect a kidney problem is by a blood test. Mature cats and cats that show any signs of early kidney disease should be screened for kidney function.

WHAT TO DO ABOUT IT

Kidney failure is sneaky. Many times, the symptoms are masked or completely invisible until the damage is critical. The typical cat in kidney failure has already lost about 70 percent of her kidney function by the time she's diagnosed. Veterinarians sometimes talk about what is called "end-stage" kidney disease when things start getting that bad. This diagnosis is just what it sounds like. Treatment for end-stage kidney disease can prolong the cat's life and make her feel better, but the end is inevitable.

This doesn't mean that every cat showing signs of kidney trouble is doomed. Sometimes, an infection can set in and the kidneys will shut down. Quick treatment can stop the infection and get the cat back on her feet with very little long-term damage.

Watch for the signs. Do you notice your cat drinking more? Has she suddenly quit eating? Is she listless or depressed? Does she seem to be urinating a lot more or barely at all? Does she seem sore over the lower part of her back or sit in a hunched-up "pain crouch"? All of these—along with vomiting and diarrhea—are signs of a possible kidney problem or infection.

Get to the vet. Home care for cats with kidney problems is only follow-up care. You need a vet to diagnose the problem, start treatment, and possibly even hospitalize your cat until she's stable.

Do the right thing. You'll probably be given a very strict diet for your cat and possibly some medications. Follow your vet's instructions as if your cat's life depends on it—because it does.

☎ WHEN TO CALL THE VET

You should call the vet immediately if any of the warning signs of kidney failure show up in your cat. Other problems have similar symptoms, and only a thorough exam and blood test can determine for sure that it's a kidney problem. The sooner you can catch it, the better the odds will be.

✳ DANGER LEVEL: Kidney failure is extremely dangerous.

Caring for the Elderly Cat

Old age catches up with all of us, humans and cats alike. We slow down, get set in our ways, and nothing works quite as well as it used to.

Signs of age happen inside and outside a geriatric cat. She'll probably drop some weight and muscle tone, giving her a gaunt "old cat" look. Her coat will probably lose some of its shine and may seem more disheveled, usually because she can't groom as well on account of losing teeth and those rough rasps on her tongue. Loss of flexibility and arthritis will slow down her pace, make jumping and climbing tougher, and make her less interested in play—and possibly more ornery when bothered.

As the internal organs wind down, her appetite and elimination will change along with her physical appearance. Your vet can tell you if these changes are within the normal range for an aging cat.

Your geriatric cat needs more peace and quiet (so don't get her a brand new kitten to "pep her up"), a diet designed for her changing needs (check with your vet or a veterinary nutritionist), and most likely more litter boxes, since the urges come on quicker and are harder to control.

LIVER DISEASE

WHAT IT IS

The liver plays an important role in metabolism and taking toxins and other unneeded compounds out of the blood. Liver damage or disease can be the result of a birth defect, infections, poisoning, or other conditions such as heart disease.

Because liver problems are often part of other illnesses, they usually don't have unique symptoms of their own. The notable exception is jaundice, which is a yellowish cast to the white of the cat's eye and possibly even her skin and under her tongue. Usually, abnormal liver function is only discovered or verified through blood tests.

WHAT TO DO ABOUT IT

Keep a sharp eye out. Liver problems due to infection and poisoning can often be stopped and much of the damage reversed if caught early enough. Watch for symptoms, and don't wait too long to call the vet if your cat is sick (especially if she's not getting better). Never assume any illness will get better by itself.

Since the clinical signs of liver disease are the same as several other illnesses it can be difficult to determine what's wrong with your cat. These signs include loss of appetite, vomiting, diarrhea, fever, weight loss, dehydration, seizures, and increased urination (thus increased water consumption). Once you notice these symptoms, check for any signs of jaundice to determine if the problem is liver-related.

Follow directions. Once a cat has been diagnosed with liver disease, her recovery depends on you. Carefully follow all diet and medication instructions your vet gives you. Resist the temptation to cheat in order to make your cat "feel better"; in the long run, you may be shortening her life.

WHEN TO CALL THE VET

Jaundice is a sure sign that something's not normal in the liver, so call the vet immediately. Since the other signs of liver disease look the same as other illnesses, the best bet is to follow the guidelines for evaluating your cat's condition as discussed in Chapter 4,

"What Every Cat Owner Should Know," and call the vet if symptoms persist.

✳ DANGER LEVEL: Liver disease is usually fatal if not treated, and some forms are fatal no matter what. Therefore, liver disease is extremely dangerous.

Obesity

What it is

Obesity is usually defined as being 15 percent or more over the average body weight for a particular individual. Since cats usually weigh somewhere between eight and ten pounds, any cat that tips the scales at more than 12 pounds is probably carrying too much weight. It's difficult to get an accurate weight on your cat at home so another way to tell is feeling the cat's ribs. You shouldn't be able to see the cat's ribs, but you should be able to feel each one under the hair and skin. As in people, a belly that protrudes much farther than the ribs is also a sign of weight gain.

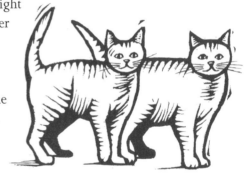

Overweight cats are at higher risk for more serious or life-threatening illnesses, including heart disease and diabetes. They are less active, which may also be an important factor in urinary tract problems like FUS (see the section on cystitis in this chapter).

What to do about it

Get 'em going. There's only one way to lose weight safely: Burn more calories than you eat. You're not going to convince your cat to get on the treadmill or the stair machine or to take up jogging, so it's up to you to increase her activity. Sometimes, introducing a young, active cat will get an obese cat moving out of self-defense, but the most reliable method is for you to exercise her with regular daily play sessions.

Less is more. A weight loss diet means cutting your cat's calories by about 30 percent until she hits the target weight, then maintaining the right number of calories to keep her at her lower weight. (This will be fewer calories than she was eating to maintain her weight.)

Cats are particularly notorious for being bad sports when they don't get as much to eat as they want (or have become used to), so be ready for some protests at first. To get your fat cat on the road to fitness, be sure to feed her less. Reducing calories means reducing the amount of food. Period.

You should also cut out snacks and treats. If you feel you absolutely must give your cat a treat, take a few morsels of food out of an already smaller meal and give it to her later. The overall calorie count (amount of food) for the day must stay down, no matter what!

Another guideline to follow is to give her lots of small meals. If your dieting cat gorges on her more humble repast and acts like she's starving three hours later, try splitting her food up into several little meals, gradually reducing the number until she's back to two or so a day.

And finally, don't "free feed" your cat. You can't tell how much your cat is eating if you leave a bowl of food out all day. Keep meals at regular intervals, and pick up what isn't eaten.

Easy does it. Your cat didn't get fat overnight or in one week. It took months or years. Gradual weight loss lets the body adjust to the changes and puts less stress on internal organs. The increase in your cat's activity will help regulate the rate of weight loss and speed things up as your cat gets fitter. Never put a cat on a starvation diet; starvation and rapid weight loss can trigger a fatal liver disease.

What about low-calorie foods? Low-cal cat foods are designed to make your cat feel full while actually giving her less calories than a full meal. In some cases, your vet may prescribe a weight-reducing food or suggest buying one of the low-cal commercial brands. In general, it's better not to change your cat's food—if you can help it—and just feed less of what she usually gets. However, switching to a low-cal food so that your cat successfully loses weight is better than keeping her on the same food—and keeping her fat.

☎ WHEN TO CALL THE VET

It's probably a good idea to talk to your vet before you begin a home weight-reduction program for your cat, just to make sure there's nothing you've overlooked. If your weight-loss program doesn't seem to be working after several weeks, you should definitely call the vet for advice. Any cat who begins looking plumper in a very short period of time needs to see the vet as soon as possible; quick weight gain can be a sign of very serious illness.

✳ DANGER LEVEL: Obesity is moderately to very dangerous, since it increases a cat's risk of life-threatening illness. The health risks go up as both the weight and the length of time that the cat remains overweight go up.

RINGWORM

WHAT IT IS

Ringworm isn't a worm, it's a skin fungus. It gets its name from the round, red, scaly patches that the fungus often causes. Cats are infamous for getting ringworm and for being carriers. A cat can actually have an active case of ringworm and have no symptoms at all. Ringworm can be spread to other cats, dogs, and even people. Also, spores from the ringworm fungus can stay active in the environment (in other words, your home) for a very long time.

Cats—and people—with weak or undeveloped immune systems are more likely to have cases of ringworm, so very young or very old cats or cats debilitated by other diseases are at the greatest risk.

Treat your cat. If you think your cat has ringworm—a safe bet when you see the "classic" round bald patches with red, scaly skin, but a distinct possibility with any kind of rash or scabs on your cat—you've got to knock out the fungus on the cat and in the home (including on other pets). Clip the hair around the scaly patches and scrub with Betadine (povidone-iodine) every day. Then use a cotton ball to apply a dilution of household bleach and water, consisting of one part bleach to 32 parts water. (Be absolutely certain to dilute first!) Over-the-counter products are also effective, with those containing miconazole or clotrimazole being the best.

If you're not sure what you're seeing is ringworm, the lesions get worse, or the outbreak spreads, get help from your vet as soon as possible. Ringworm is usually a self-limiting problem, meaning that is goes only so far and then stops of its own accord; but if it gets out of control, it can be around for a long time and keep coming back.

Treat all your pets. Most likely, all your cats and dogs (if you have them), as well as the infected cat, will need at least an antifungal bath. In some cases, your vet may recommend an oral medication for the affected cat and possibly for other animals as a preventative or to knock out spores on carriers.

Treat the home. Wash all pet bedding, toys, and bowls in hot water. If it can't be washed or disinfected, discard it in an outdoor trash can. Thoroughly vacuum all floors and furniture and discard the vacuum bag immediately in an outdoor location. Disinfect uncarpeted floors and other hard surfaces in rooms where the cat goes with the diluted bleach solution. Cleaning and disinfecting must be repeated at least weekly until the cat is completely free of all signs of ringworm. It's a good idea to do a disinfection from time to time after that, since ringworm spores can survive in your home for years.

An ounce of prevention. Cats who don't go outdoors and aren't exposed to other cats rarely have ringworm. Keep your cat indoors and use in-home pet sitters instead of boarding and you most likely will not have to deal with a ringworm outbreak.

☎ WHEN TO CALL THE VET

Since ringworm is persistent, sometimes hard to diagnose without special equipment, and cats can carry it without symptoms, veterinary assistance is always a good idea. Lesions that don't heal, look infected, get worse, spread rapidly, or don't respond to home treatment are either something other than ringworm or a very hot case of ringworm that's gotten out of control. Either way, call your vet.

✳ DANGER LEVEL: Ringworm is persistent and a nuisance but not dangerous. Cats and people with suppressed immune systems (from chemotherapy or AIDS, for example) can have extremely serious outbreaks that can become infected; ringworm for these individuals is moderately dangerous.

SCRAPES AND SCRATCHES

WHAT THEY ARE

Abrasions (scrapes and scratches) are damage to the outer layers of skin. The most common cause of scrapes and scratches in cats is other cats. Usually, cats keep their claws retracted during play, and their thick hair protects them from accidental nicks. Vigorous play, a miscalculation, or an unplayful smack can cause an abrasion, usually most noticeable around the ears and face where the hair is more sparse. Unaltered cats and cats who go outdoors are more likely to get into out-and-out fights and suffer bite and scratch wounds.

What to do about them

Keep it clean. For fresh scratches simple soap-and-water cleanup, using a washcloth or cotton ball, is usually enough first aid. Don't try to prevent your cat from licking a scratch—that's Mother Nature's way of taking care of it, and she knows what she's doing. But do keep an eye on your cat. Occasionally, a cat may overdo it and require some type of restraint to prevent mutilation of the wound.

Look for more. Ruffle through your cat's fur and check for additional scratches. A veterinarian from an animal shelter remarks, "Any time we had to shave a stray cat with visible scratches for surgery, we found more scratches or scars all over her body."

Plumb the depths. How deep is the wound? Anything that bleeds noticeably needs more attention than a simple scratch. First, stop the bleeding with direct pressure, using a cotton ball or gauze. (You may need help restraining the cat.) Trim the hair from around the edge of the wound, and wash thoroughly with soap and water. Bandaging usually isn't necessary, and most scratches, scrapes, and minor wounds heal better and faster in the open air. Just be sure to keep the wound area clean.

When to call the vet

Any serious wound or wound that won't stop bleeding needs immediate veterinary attention. If direct pressure doesn't stop bleeding in a couple minutes—or if the wound is spurting blood—your cat is in grave danger. Take your cat directly to the vet, and continue to apply pressure and bandages until you can get her there.

Bite wounds should be treated by a vet, too, since they can become infected easily. Sometimes bites or other wounds will close up with some dirt or germs inside, causing an abscess—a painful, swollen pocket of infection. If the site of a wound swells, leaks pus, or is sensitive to the touch, or if your cat suddenly begins to run a fever, call your vet right away.

✳ DANGER LEVEL: Most minor scrapes and scratches are not dangerous; deep wounds require veterinary attention.

Seizure

What it is

Seizure, or convulsion, is a catchall word used to describe sudden attacks of changes in behavior that include loss of consciousness, loss of motor control (staggering, falling down, poor coordination), and loss of bladder or bowel control. Seizures can be so mild as to be almost unnoticeable (the cat walks a bit strangely or acts "spacey" for a few minutes and then is fine) to frighteningly severe (the cat staggers, falls down, voids bladder and bowels, loses consciousness, and goes stiff).

Nervous system disorders, injuries (especially to the head), concussions, poisoning, tumors, stroke, infection, and high fever are just some of the causes of seizures. Epilepsy is a recurring seizure disorder in which a malfunction of the nervous system causes the brain to "misfire" messages to the body. These "misfired" messages result in a seizure.

A frequent concern voiced about seizure victims is that they may swallow their tongue and suffocate. While an unconscious or semiconscious cat should be kept on her side to prevent the tongue from sliding to the back of the throat and partially obstructing the breathing passage, it's physically impossible for a normally attached tongue to be swallowed. Sometimes, injury or an allergic reaction to a food, medicine, or insect bite (anaphylaxis) can cause the tongue to swell and prevent breathing. This is a dire emergency, and veterinary medical care is needed immediately.

What to do about it

Keep her in one place. Witnessing a cat having a seizure is frightening. Being the cat is even more frightening. She needs you to stay calm and keep her under gentle restraint so she doesn't injure herself. Unfortunately, she doesn't know she needs you to do that, so put a fluffy towel or light blanket over the cat to restrain her; any cat will bite or scratch, often severely, when in seizure. Don't try to stop the involuntary jerking movements that go with some seizures since you can hurt the cat. Talk to her in soothing tones; even if she seems to be unresponsive, she may be able to hear you (and it will help to steady your nerves).

Watch the time. The first time it happens, a seizure seems to go on forever. However, most really only last a minute or two before the cat starts coming out of it. If the seizure doesn't show signs of letting up after two minutes (or if it passes but recurs again in less than 24 hours), you have an emergency on your hands—get to the vet.

Get to the root. Even if your cat recovers quickly from a seizure, make an appointment with the vet to try and figure out the cause. Seizure can be the result of tumors, hypoglycemia, nutritional deficiencies, or epilepsy—all of which can usually be treated or controlled.

When to call the vet

A seizure that doesn't begin to let up after a minute or two, lets up but then comes on again, or recurs in less than 24 hours is a serious symptom and needs immediate veterinary care. Cats who have seizures that let up quickly and from which the cat fully recovers should be seen by the vet as soon as possible.

✳ DANGER LEVEL: Although frightening, a seizure that begins easing up within two minutes is only moderately dangerous. However, continuous or multiple seizures can be extremely dangerous.

Spraying

What it is

Urine spraying to mark territory is a common behavior in cats. Mature unaltered males do it most typically, but neutered males and even spayed females may also show the behavior. The cat backs up to a vertical surface, standing with tail erect. Urine is sprayed on the surface with a characteristic jiggling of the tail and sometimes treading with the back feet.

What to do about it

Get to the bottom of it. Urine spraying may be a sign of physical maturity in a male kitten, a signal that there's either a physical problem with the urinary tract, or a behavioral problem that needs prompt attention. Don't assume it's just a behavioral problem though; if a physical problem is the original cause, no amount of behavior modification will help. On the other hand, the longer the physical problem goes untreated, the more ingrained the habit of spraying becomes and the harder it will be to break (if you can at all) once the physical cause is removed. Have your cat thoroughly examined by your veterinarian. If everything checks out normally, it's probably a behavior problem. Follow the advice in the section on spraying in Chapter 8, "Common Behavorial Problems and Home Remedies."

"Fix" the problem. When male cats reach sexual maturity, they often announce it by beginning to mark their territory—your home—by spraying urine. Mature tomcat urine is especially pungent, so you'd be well advised to nip this behavior in the bud by neutering male kittens by the age of six months (unless your veterinarian recommends waiting longer). Some humane organizations now promote or practice early neuter or spay, altering kittens as young as seven weeks old. Preliminary studies show no major problems with cats neutered younger than six months of age, and the kittens recover amazingly fast.

Girls will be boys. Sometimes, a spayed female cat will begin spraying, although females aren't especially known for marking territory that way. The reduction in female hormones after spaying is suspected as the culprit, and your vet may recommend hormone therapy as a way of breaking the habit. In fact, female hormones may be used with neutered male cats who spray, for the same reason.

☎ WHEN TO CALL THE VET

Make an appointment with your vet as soon as your cat starts spraying. Remember, the sooner you find or rule out a physical cause, the more likely you are to change the behavior. If your cat shows spraying behavior but produces no urine, watch to see if he urinates in the litter box. If so, consider yourself lucky—he's just going through the motions. However, if he produces no urine in the litter box, produces frequent small amounts, or cries in pain while attempting to urinate or spray, he could have a urinary blockage. This is a life-or-death emergency that needs immediate veterinary attention.

✳ DANGER LEVEL: Spraying is a tremendous nuisance but not dangerous. However, inappropriate urination is perhaps the most common reason owners surrender their cats to animal shelters or have otherwise healthy cats euthanized.

TICKS

WHAT THEY ARE

Ticks are small, blood-sucking insects that attach themselves to warm-blooded animals by burying their mouth parts into the skin. Once a tick begins to feed, its body expands, often to many times normal. A gorged tick may look like a small mole or roundish bump of odd-colored flesh. Ticks are usually found on vegetation, several feet off the ground, and drop onto passing animals such as your cat or dog.

Because their mouth parts make contact with the blood stream of the host, ticks can transmit diseases, most notably Lyme disease. It's important, then, that ticks be removed as soon as possible—and with their entire body intact. The longer the tick is imbedded, the greater the risk of spreading anything it might be carrying, and any part of the tick left behind could still contain infectious matter.

What to do about it

Keep out of the country. Cats that remain indoors almost never get ticks, unless they're carried in by other pets, people, or rodent pests. Even if your cat goes outdoors in a "controlled" way (on a handheld leash, for example), keep her away from tall grass and out from under bushes and shrubs—anywhere ticks could be lurking, waiting to drop.

The best defense is a strong offense. If your cat goes outdoors, regularly dust or spray her with a flea and tick product containing pyrethrins (a natural insecticide found in flowers from the mum family). Rodents often carry ticks, so eliminating rodent populations and nesting sites from your home and property will cut down on the number of ticks, too.

> Ticks bite people, too, and can cause Lyme disease and Rocky Mountain spotted fever.

Nice and easy does it. Check your cat for ticks any time she goes outdoors, especially in more suburban and rural settings and during warmer weather. If you find a tick on your cat's body, it's important to remove it quickly. The best way to do this is to grasp the tick at the skin line with a pair of forceps or tweezers. Try to grab the tick as close to its head as possible and pull gently and steadily straight out from the cat's body. Forget what you may have learned about burning ticks out; it doesn't work well, and you run the risk of badly singeing or burning your cat.

It ain't over 'til it's over. Ticks are hardy creatures. When you remove one, don't assume it's dead or that you'll be rid of it by throwing it in the garbage or sending it down the drain or toilet. They can crawl back out from any of these destinations, ready to attach themselves to the next mammal that happens by. Throwing them outdoors gets them out of your house but may just be passing the problem along to someone else. It's best to put the removed tick immediately into a small jar with rubbing alcohol or insecticide, and then seal the jar securely. This method not only ensures the demise of the little pest and seals off any escape, it preserves the insect in case the tick bite victim develops complications.

Watch for complications. Once you remove a tick from your cat, keep a close eye on her for the next week or so. Ticks can carry some serious diseases, so contact your vet at the first sign of sickness, especially fever, loss of appetite, listlessness, or apparent stiffness or aching in the joints. Sometimes the tick bite itself can cause a progressive weakness in the back legs of the cat, a condition called tick-bite paralysis. This usually clears up on its own, once the tick is removed.

☎ WHEN TO CALL THE VET

Contact your veterinarian if your cat shows any signs of illness within a week or so after you remove a tick, or if any redness or swelling develops at the bite location. Ticks are small and can be easily missed, so be particularly aware of symptoms any time your cat goes outdoors—even if you don't see any ticks.

✻ DANGER LEVEL: Because ticks carry some diseases, tick bites should be considered moderately dangerous; however, in areas where Lyme disease is prevalent, tick bites should be treated as dangerous.

Tooth and Gum Problems

What they are

Just like people, cats have a set of baby (deciduous) teeth when young, which are replaced by permanent teeth. Similarly, keeping the teeth and gums healthy requires regular preventative care. Food and saliva form plaque, which can mineralize into hard deposits of tartar. Gingivitis (inflammation of the gums) and loss of permanent teeth can result. Actual cavities are relatively rare, but pitting and other tooth damage can result from neglecting oral hygiene. Mouth pain and tooth loss may reduce a cat's interest or ability to eat, causing weight loss and making the cat more prone to illness.

What to do about it

Brush regularly. You don't need to have an actual toothbrush and paste, but giving your cat's teeth a good going-over a few times a week is the best way to fight plaque. There are pet toothbrushes available, but you can also just use a piece of gauze or rough cloth that is moistened and wrapped around your index finger. Rub the cloth vigorously over the outside surfaces of the teeth (you don't usually need to get the inner or biting surfaces). This will help keep your cat's teeth clean and gums healthy.

Give Tabby the crunchies. Hard, dry cat food is the best bet to prevent plaque and tartar. If you can convince your cat to chew rawhide or a hard rubber dog toy, that can help, too—although many cats refuse them. There are now some chew-toy products on the market made especially for cats.

Look out for tartar. Plaque is a mushy whitish material that you can easily scrape off the teeth with your fingernail. Tartar, on the other hand, is greyish, white, or brown and does not come off with brushing. Tartar buildup needs to be removed by your vet.

Gums the word. Giving your cat a weekly gum massage helps keep gums healthy and prevent tooth loss. Using a cotton swab, rub the area where the teeth and gums meet. If the gums are red or there's any bleeding, it could be gingivitis, and your cat may need veterinary treatment.

> Cats don't have wisdom teeth. Instead, the four longest teeth rest in the corners of the mouth.

Broken teeth and abscesses. A cracked canine tooth isn't rare in cats, especially outdoor cats and former strays. Broken teeth are usually only a problem if the pulp (the capsule of blood vessels and nerves in the middle of the tooth) is exposed. This can be quite painful, and the tooth may die. In either case, there's a risk of infection in the tooth root—an abscess. Abscesses can also form from bad oral hygiene. Symptoms include swelling around the mouth that may come and go and tenderness. Broken teeth that have exposed pulp, die, or abscess need to be removed by your veterinarian.

☎ WHEN TO CALL THE VET

Make an appointment with your vet if your cat has tartar buildup, shows signs of gingivitis (red or bleeding gums), has a broken tooth with exposed pulp or that has died (it will usually become discolored), has any swelling or tenderness around the mouth, or has any loose permanent teeth. Adult cats often lose teeth as they get older—especially the small front incisors—and veterinary care usually isn't necessary for this.

✳ DANGER LEVEL: Tooth and gum problems can cause discomfort, make the cat touchy, and give her bad breath—annoying but not particularly dangerous. However, as the problems worsen, infections can set in or the cat can stop eating altogether and should be considered dangerous if not treated.

UPPER RESPIRATORY DISEASES (FELINE "COLDS")

WHAT THEY ARE

Coughing, sneezing, runny eyes and nose, and possibly a fever are all the familiar symptoms of a cold. Unlike in humans, however, most feline "colds" have known (and preventable) causes, usually one of three kinds of viruses. Safe and reliable vaccines are available to prevent them all.

Even vaccinated cats may have upper respiratory infections, though, and most will resolve within a few days to two weeks. Severe infections or those in cats with weakened immune systems may last several weeks. Although antibiotics won't kill the viruses, they are often prescribed to treat or prevent secondary infections that take hold when the virus damages tissue in the nose, eyes, sinuses, mouth, and possibly even the lungs of an affected cat.

Early signs of upper respiratory disease include sneezing, watery eyes, and a clear discharge from the nose. The cat usually runs a fever and may salivate. As the infection advances, the lining of the eyes may get inflamed (conjunctivitis), giving the eyes a "meaty" appearance; the nasal discharge contains pus; the tearing from the eyes turns white; and ulcers may appear in the mouth or on the tongue. Advanced symptoms—most commonly seen if the disease is left untreated— include the eyelid being glued shut by pus and discharge with ulceration and destruction of the eyeball, loss of appetite due to obstruction of the nose by mucous and pus, and pneumonia. Viral pneumonia can be fatal and about one in five cats that develop it will die.

What to do about it

Be sure she has her shots. Current vaccinations are the best protection against upper respiratory viruses. Even indoor cats who never have contact with another cat need their shots since the viruses are carried through the air.

Don't wait for it to go away. Even though many upper respiratory infections clear up on their own, don't assume this one will. Notify your vet. The virus can attack the eyeball, causing permanent damage or blindness. Also, a cat with an untreated cold will stop eating or may develop a fatal case of pneumonia.

Don't spread it around. Upper respiratory viruses are highly contagious. A cat with an active case must be kept away from other cats. Wash your hands thoroughly with soap and hot water after petting, medicating, or otherwise working with the sick cat.

When to call the vet

If you call the vet when you see the early symptoms of a cold, the odds are you can prevent the worst-case scenario. Veterinarians can recommend a vaccine that can prevent feline "colds." This vaccination may not always work, but it can improve your cat's chances for a healthy recovery. At any rate, once any of the later symptoms appear (pus in the discharge from nose or eyes, ulcers in the mouth or on the tongue, loss of appetite), get the cat to the vet immediately.

DANGER LEVEL: Upper respiratory infections are fairly common and mild ones are only moderately dangerous. However, if left untreated or found in very young or elderly cats or cats with weakened immune systems, complications from what started out as a simple cold can be fatal.

Vomiting

What it is

Vomiting means that the contents of the stomach or intestines are ejected through the mouth. This should not be confused with regurgitation, which is the ejection of the contents of the esophagus (the swallowing tube of the throat) and the pharynx (the space where the back of the mouth meets the top of the esophagus and windpipe). Regurgitation means that the expelled material has not made it all the way to the stomach and could be a sign of a problem in the mouth, pharynx, or esophagus.

Anyone who has a cat knows that vomiting isn't an uncommon thing. When accompanied by other signs of illness, it can be an important early warning or a symptom of serious trouble. A cat that vomits once or twice—without any other symptoms like fever, persistent diarrhea, weakness, or pain in the abdomen—probably just has an upset tummy from what (or how much) she ate and can be safely treated at home.

What to do about it

Slow down the chowing down. Reflex vomiting happens when a cat bolts down her food in too much of a hurry. Cats rescued from the outdoors are notorious for "stray syndrome"; they still believe they have to gobble up as much food as they can in as short a time as possible. The result is often the whole thing coming back up again. There are several ways to slow down the pace.

- Reduce competition from other pets. The mere presence of other animals at mealtime encourages a chowhound cat to gobble her food, since she may feel the need to get as much food in while she can. Be sure she has her own food bowl and gets fed at predictable mealtimes. Feed her in a separate room, if possible.

- Feed your cat less but more often. Several small meals during the day will often stay down better than gorging on two or three big ones. Also, consider changing the type of food you feed your cat. The faster the food goes down, the faster a chowhound cat will eat. Soft food can be swallowed as quickly as the cat can get it into her mouth. A good crunchy, dry food has to be chewed up, which slows down her eating.

- Take a look at what's in your cat's food. Pet food or food additives can disagree with cats' tummies. Keep track of when your cat vomits. Is it usually after eating a certain kind, brand, or type of food? She may like fish, for example, but it may not like her. The eye-catching cat food with the bright colors may have dyes she's allergic to. And the stuff that looks like chunks of meat may have additives she can't digest well.

What doesn't go down, can't come up. Fast your cat for at least 12 hours (but no more than 24) to give her stomach time to settle and her system time to clear out whatever is disagreeing with her. Break the fast with a small meal of bland, easy-to-digest food such as turkey or chicken baby food. Look for the pureed—not the chunky—kind and get the "beginner" or "first" baby food. If she keeps that down for a few hours, give her another small meal, continuing with more every few hours as long as the vomiting doesn't start again. The next day, try giving her full-size meals at the regular times, but use bland foods. (Try the "quiet diet" suggested in the diarrhea section of this chapter.)

Keep her hydrated. It's important to make sure your cat is getting enough water, especially since she's not getting any from her food. If she has loose stools with the vomiting, she's losing even more fluid. However, an upset stomach can be irritated even by being full of water, so limit how much she can drink at a time. Try putting a single ice cube in the water bowl (you can crush it if you prefer) to ensure she only drinks small amounts. Replace the cube when the bowl is empty.

Make the medicine fit the problem. Vomiting isn't a disease in and of itself; it's a signal that something else is wrong. It could be as simple as a cat eating too fast or as serious as liver or kidney disease. You should never continue a home treatment if vomiting persists for more than a day, doesn't improve after 24 hours of home treatment, or is accompanied by other signs of disease. Some over-the-counter stomach remedies are safe and effective for cats, particularly those with magnesium hydroxide or magnesium aluminum (products like Milk of Magnesia or Kaopectate). Make sure you call your vet to get the correct dosage.

Look for a foreign invasion. An alien horde in your cat's stomach or intestines—in other words, worms or other parasites—is a common cause of vomiting. Cats are also curious creatures and will eat things we would find unappetizing or downright disgusting. Although sometimes those strange food items just make Tabby sick, other times the cat can swallow a nonfood item that gets stuck in the esophagus, stomach, or intestine. These "foreign bodies" must be removed by your veterinarian, sometimes requiring surgery.

☎ WHEN TO CALL THE VET

A cat who vomits repeatedly, retches repeatedly without producing anything substantial, shows blood in the vomit, or has projectile vomiting (the material is expelled with great force) should go to the vet immediately. If your cat has other signs of illness—especially fever, weakness, depression, or a painful or swollen belly—call your vet right away, even if the cat has only vomited once or twice.

✳ DANGER LEVEL: The major risks involved with vomiting are dehydration, weight loss, and, if the cat vomits regularly over a long period of time, malnutrition. A single incident of vomiting is not dangerous, if it occurs with no other symptoms. Vomiting that persists or is accompanied by other signs of disease is dangerous to extremely dangerous, depending on the cause.

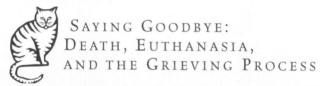

SAYING GOODBYE: DEATH, EUTHANASIA, AND THE GRIEVING PROCESS

Pet owners (and veterinarians) have a unique responsibility: We can often choose when it's time for an animal companion to die. Euthanasia means "good death," a controlled way to end an animal's life almost instantaneously and painlessly.

Veterinarians have an ethical obligation to end an animal's suffering when death is unavoidable and the cat is in obvious pain. But the vet can't give your cat that final needle unless you say so. For some cat owners, that's a decision that weighs too heavily on their shoulders, and they decide to wait and see if there will be a miracle or to just "let nature take its course." Of course, once in awhile there is a miraculous recovery, but most of the time the end is the same—and the cat suffers longer. While the burden of the decision can be overwhelming, ultimately, the cat's quality of life must be the most important consideration.

Whether the cat dies of old age or illness or is euthanized, it's important that the owner understands that grief at the loss of a beloved pet is a natural and normal response. Seek out support from friends and family who understand your attachment, or check with your local humane society for pet loss support groups in your area. (For pet loss support hotlines, see Chapter 9, "Where to Learn More.") Resist the temptation to go out and replace your departed companion immediately—she can't be replaced. Give yourself time to grieve and recover from your loss.

Worms

What They Are

Your cat's stomach and intestines are home to a host of tiny creatures—microscopic critters that are actually normal, natural, and healthy for her. But sometimes the eggs of parasites get into her digestive system, developing into adult worms or other things that feed off the food going through her gut and steal its nutrition. Worms will thrive in the cat's gut, producing more eggs that are shed in the cat's feces and spread to other hosts.

The most common unwanted tenants of your cat's digestive tract are roundworms, tapeworms, and Coccidia. Roundworms (or ascarids) look like short strands of thick white thread, and a cat with a particularly bad case may actually vomit some up. Adult roundworms lay eggs, which are passed in the cat's stool, and can be seen under a microscope. Tapeworms attach to the lining of the cat's intestine by their heads (called the scolex) and grow by segments. Each segment contains eggs, ripens, and is shed with the cat's stool. Since the eggs are contained in the segments, microscopic examination of a stool sample may not find them. Sometimes, the tapeworm segments—which look like grains of rice—can be found clinging to the cat's rectum. Coccidia aren't actually worms but microscopic one-celled organisms that live and breed in the cat's intestines.

What To Do About It

Vanquish the vectors. Your cat has to get worms from somewhere or something else. A vector is the fancy word for the thing she gets it from. Fleas, for example, carry tapeworm. A cat with fleas grooms herself, swallows the flea with the tapeworm eggs, and—voila! Similarly, a cat who shares a litter box (or goes outdoors) where a cat already infected with worms goes is likely to come in contact with eggs or spores shed in the infected cat's stool and—voila! Another common vector is infected birds, mice, or other unfortunates that your cat captures and eats. Cats who hunt or are used as "mousers" are more likely to pick up parasites of many kinds, including toxoplasmosis, which has some health concerns for humans (see the section on zoonotic diseases in Chapter 4, "What Every Cat Owner Should Know").

No news may not be good news. Kittens with worms may show diarrhea, slow weight gain, and a pot belly, and adult cats may have dark tarry stool, vomiting, diarrhea, and weight loss—or no signs at all. Just because your cat doesn't have any symptoms doesn't mean she doesn't have worms. If your cat has never been checked for worms, it's a good idea to do it and to have a stool sample checked for any new cat brought into your home. Even if your cat has been treated for worms, should she get fleas, go outdoors, or hunt mice or other small creatures regularly, it's almost a sure bet she's got them again.

Only rely on the good stuff. Over-the-counter worming medications don't have enough punch to knock out worms for good. No home or folk remedies have been shown to be both effective and safe enough to get the job done, either. Prevention is the best cure, but if your cat does have worms, get the right medication in the right doses from your veterinarian.

Soothe the symptoms. Even after your cat has been treated for worms—and sometimes as a result of the treatment—she may have some stomach or intestinal distress. Following the steps in this chapter for treating diarrhea and vomiting can make her more comfortable while her gut gets back to normal.

☎ WHEN TO CALL THE VET

All cats should have a stool sample examined for worms—the earlier the better. While many cats who have worms may have no symptoms, an infestation that goes unchecked for months or years has been robbing your cat of nutrients. What's more, she's been shedding the worms' eggs in her stool, passing them along to other animals in the house and in some cases, even to people.

Even if a cat has been wormed in the past, the treatment is not effective for life—it just kills the worms that are in the cat's body at that time. Cats who go outdoors, hunt, are fed (or eat) raw or undercooked meat or meat products (including organs), have fleas, or share quarters with a cat who has been diagnosed with worms have probably been reinfected and should have a stool sample checked.

✳ DANGER LEVEL: The most common worms are usually not danger- ous, although untreated cases—especially in debilitated cats—can be dangerous. Some of the rarer types of worms and one-celled parasites can be moderately dangerous to dangerous, depending on how quickly they're diagnosed and treated.

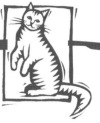

Behavior and Training

Although it may seem like a contradiction in terms, you can train a cat—and should. Having a well-socialized cat has many benefits: It's easier to get him to the vet or the groomer; home health care and prevention go easier; and people will actually want to come to your home without fear of being scratched, bitten, or having themselves or their belongings anointed with various feline bodily fluids.

These next pages will introduce you to the mysteries of feline behavior and provide you with tried-and-true tips for shaping your cat into a decent citizen, although probably not a model one—that may be asking too much of any cat.

Understanding Cat Behavior

There are so many fascinating ways that cats communicate with each other. Some of their methods are so subtle that we humans are not sensitive enough to understand what they are saying. Cats often use mild and controlled signs of body language. A minor flick of the tail or the slightest movement of the ears send messages that are worth a thousand words to another cat. But since their body language is so restrained, we often find it difficult to comprehend, so we end up making mistakes trying to interpret their messages. It's easier for us to discern what cats are saying when they use their voices. Their range of sounds—from a gentle purr to a seething hiss—let us know if a cat is happy or angry. Once we learn to make sense of the body language and the vocalizations of cats, we are one step closer to understanding cat behavior.

Nature or Nurture?

In the study of behavior, experts talk about nature versus nurture, meaning which behaviors are inbred (or instinct) and which are learned. It's an argument that will probably never be completely settled. Most experts agree, however, that animals like cats and dogs have both kinds of behavior; they just disagree on which ones are which—and which kind is more important.

An example of an instinctual behavior would be what happens when you run your hand down the cat's back, from his head to his tail. That response of sticking his backside up in the air is hardwired into his nervous system. A learned behavior is something like your cat running into the kitchen whenever he hears the can opener. That is, if you've ever fed him anything out of a can.

Reflex actions. Classical animal behavior talks about reflexes and has its own nature versus nurture debate. Unconditioned reflexes are those the body seems to produce on its own. For example, if you kick your leg up when the doctor taps your knee with a rubber hammer. A conditioned reflex is a learned response. Most of us have heard of Pavlov's dog, who was trained to know that food was coming whenever he heard a bell ring. After awhile, Doc Pavlov could ring the bell and his dog would start salivating—even if there was no food present.

The great debate resolved. Actually, even Pavlov had to admit that his conditioned dog didn't have a completely learned response. If there wasn't an instinctive response of salivating in the presence of food to begin with, Pavlov could never have trained the dog to do it when he heard the bell. What Pavlov really proved was that animals are born with a set of instinctive, natural behaviors, and they learn how to apply and adapt them as needed.

What it all means for your cat. In order to train your cat, you need to understand his behavior. You'll never get him to do anything that's totally outside of his natural behaviors, but you can teach him how to adapt those behaviors so that both of you live happily ever after.

The best example is the litter box: Cats have the instinctive behavior of digging in loose materials and burying their urine and feces. As long as the litter box is the place that appeals to the cat most, that's where he'll consistently eliminate. However, he may be more intrigued by soil in your potted palm, the loose, fluffy pile of your carpeting, or the nice, soft pile of socks left in a corner of the utility room. As long as the behavior is shaped toward the litter box, you've got no problem. (See the section on litter box accidents in Chapter 8, "Common Behavioral Problems and Home Remedies.")

Speaking Feline

Obviously, cats don't have a spoken language like we do. But they do have a voice, and they make sounds that have different meanings. This is their means of communication. "Speaking feline" not only means understanding cats' vocalizations but also understanding the more complex language of cats—body language.

Cat "speech." Cats make a variety of sounds that have been given colorful and descriptive names. Their purpose can range from expressing contentment to a call for help, from solicitation of food or companionship to a blood-curdling expression of stark terror.

The classic cat sound (or vocalization) is the meow. Newborn kittens will meow with surprising volume. These vocalizations are probably to indicate hunger or cold and to help the mother cat locate them. As the cat gets older, the meow is still used largely to solicit or attract attention (for example, if your cat wants to signal you that he feels it's time for dinner).

An angry, frightened, or aggressive cat may hiss, which is a clear warning that whoever or whatever is approaching should come no closer. Hissing is often accompanied by a yowl, a throaty warning sound that rises and falls. An extremely frightened or angry cat will scream—a sound that needs no further explanation.

Calling or yodeling is that mournful, slightly spooky sound your cat makes (usually in the middle of the night) while wandering around the house. New cat owners (and even some veteran ones) sometimes mistake this normal vocalization for pain, confusion, or loneliness, assuming that their cat is in distress. Female cats in heat (estrus) yodel to signal their readiness to mate. The tomcat calls to the female to advertise his availability in a loud voice called caterwauling. This call also serves the purpose of warning rival males of his amorous intentions.

Behavior and Training

> A hiss is really a force of hot air, used by the cat to express fear and anger.

Three sounds are unique to cats. The chortle, a happy greeting sound, sounds a lot like a quick, high-pitched chuckle. There's also that strange chirping or chattering noise cats make that's usually reserved for when they see birds outside the window. This is the elusive wacka-wacka, a term coined by famed cat cartoonist B. Kliban. Finally, the purr is, of course, the most sublime of all feline sounds. It's also one of the most hotly debated. While a supremely contented cat will purr loudly, so will an extremely nervous or stressed one. This leads some researchers to think cats do it to reassure themselves. It's not even completely clear how cats purr. Most of the wild members of the cat family purr, but the household variety of cat is about the only one that can make the sound on both the exhale and the inhale.

Read my hips. The lithe, often silent movements of a cat actually speak volumes. Every inch of your cat, from the nose to the tip of the tail, communicates something.

We can think of the cat's state of mind as being more inward, more outward, or somewhere in between. A cat that is being defensive is more inward and will usually only attack if pursued. On the other hand, a cat that is ready to launch an offensive attack is more outward. The ears are a good marker of the how inward or outward a cat is feeling: The farther back the ears are laid, the more inward the cat's state of mind. This also means a curious or friendly cat will have his ears pricked (forward and erect), since those are both outward states of mind.

Wide-open eyes are an outward sign. Other body and vocal signals will tell you if it's a good kind of outward, meaning that a happy or playful cat will have wide-open eyes but so will a terrified cat. Relaxed, open eyes reflect a more neutral internal state; relaxed, narrowed eyes usually means the cat's submissive, but it could also indicate a contented cat.

The size of the cat's pupils also offer a clue to his feelings: Dilated pupils may indicate fear while constricted pupils suggest aggressive feelings. A direct stare is an outward sign, meaning, "Back off, buster!"

Even the position of a cat's mouth says something about his feelings. The more open the mouth, usually the more outward the cat's state of mind. Again, this can be rage (lips drawn back, tense) or play (lips not drawn back, relaxed). Of course, if a cat also opens his mouth wide to hiss, spit, and show sharp teeth, it is definitely an indication of anger.

A cat's tail serves many purposes, with one of them being an indicator of what a cat is saying. An erect tail is an outward sign, usually part of a friendly greeting or a "follow-me" message—watch a mother cat leading her kittens, or check out your cat the next time he tries to lure you toward where the cat food is stored. A lashing tail shows agitation, which may mean anger, excitement, or anticipation, especially just before pouncing in play or hunting. A bristled tail indicates fear, while a relaxed, gently swishing tail suggests contentment.

> Over 20 muscles control the position of a cat's ears, and this position often indicates the mood of your cat.

Body orientation is another indicator of inward or outward behavior. A straight-on approach is friendly, confident, or aggressive. When a cat makes himself

Behavior and Training

bigger, by standing taller over another cat, climbing higher, or "puffing up" his hair, it's usually a display of dominance or aggression or an outright threat. This strategy is played out in the familiar "Halloween cat" posture (sometimes called spidering or arching), where the cat turns sideways, arches his back, puffs up his hair, and hisses. This posture combines defensive elements (such as turning sideways) with clear threats (such as making himself look larger).

On the other hand, when a cat makes himself smaller, by scrunching down, rolling to his side, or leaning away, he's trying to show that he's not a threat.

AGGRESSION AND PLAY

When a cat becomes destructive, the owner is often shocked to hear the professional advice: Get a second cat. The owner's understandable concern is that two cats will do twice as much damage, and the destructive cat will now have another cat to shred. Fortunately, the former is rarely true, mostly because the cat's energy is focused on another cat. This also seems to make the latter a valid fear. There must be a period of introduction, and some hissing and minor scuffles are normal. However, many multiple-cat owners witness normal vigorous feline play and are convinced the cats still aren't getting along.

Play we must. Play is an instinctive behavior. All mammals—including cats, dogs, and people—play. While play is more frequent and energetic in younger animals, adults play as well. In fact, play persists throughout an animal's lifetime.

We must ... but why? For decades, animal behaviorists have argued that play—like all instinctive behaviors—must have some deeper reason behind it. Citing the theory of natural selection, they say that if play behavior was completely frivolous, it would be a waste of time and energy and would have been eradicated over time. Clearly, these researchers need to get out and have fun more often.

Play may well serve as practice for important adult behaviors, which is why so much of it looks like aggression. So when one cat hunkers down, twitches his backside, lashes his tail, and then pounces on his feline roommate, landing full on the unsuspecting victim's back and seizing his neck in his jaws, it's definitely play; the real-life use of that sequence of behavior is stalking and killing prey. But researchers are finally, grudgingly admitting that play could have another purpose, one which humans have known about for time immemorial: It's fun!

> Cats start playing at the age of four weeks, and the games continue the rest of their lives.

How do I know when it's for real? Feline play is often no-holds-barred: noisy running, hot pursuit, pouncing, stalking, slamming bodies, wrestling, biting, the works. But in terms of vocalization, it's relatively quiet. An out-and-out catfight would include all the same behaviors as a fun bout of play but with lots of loud hissing, yowling, screaming, and flying fur. Play uses the same behaviors as aggression, but they are inhibited: There are smacks to the head but with claws retracted; bites but with relaxed jaws and exaggerated movements.

Behavior and Training

Other hallmarks of play include frequent changes in who's the aggressor—who's on top in the wrestling match, who's chasing whom, or whose body language is more inward or outward—and the play face (a relaxed, open jaw and wide-open eyes). If you doubt that humans use the play face just watch a bunch of school children heading out the door for recess!

Bring out the best. Now that you can recognize play behavior in your cat, you can make him happier and healthier by encouraging it. If there's only one cat in the home, you have the responsibility of being his playmate. Cat toys are fine as long as they're safe (see the section on good toys and bad toys in Chapter 3, "An Ounce of Prevention"), but your cat also needs you to play with him. Chasing, stalking, and pouncing games are at the top of the feline hit parade. Cats see moving edges better than stationary ones, so toys that wiggle, bounce, roll, or bob are particularly intriguing.

Even in multiple-cat households, the humans need to play with the cats. Play is a kind of "social glue," and the more your cats recognize humans as potential playmates, the better socialized to people they will be.

> Play fighting between kittens tones muscles, develops social skills, and also teaches them the important life lesson of how to inhibit their bite.

TRAINING YOUR CAT

The cat is a very independent animal, and many cat owners will tell you that it is this independence that makes the cat such a comfortable companion around the house. Cats are not as demanding of attention as dogs. And, unlike dogs, most cats don't make any particular effort to win your approval—they'll often wait for you to come to them rather than run around trying to catch your eye.

All this means that the cat is a very easy going creature who is polite and self-possessed. But it also means that it can be difficult to train a cat. If you and your cat don't see eye to eye over a certain kind of behavior, you might have a hard time getting him to do things your way. However, don't give up hope—it's not completely impossible to modify your cat's behavior.

GETTING A CAT TO CHANGE HIS WAYS

Can a cat be trained? Surprisingly, the answer is a resounding "Yes!"—but it has to be done on feline terms. Everything in this chapter up to this point is background information, designed to help you see the world from your cat's perspective, which is an important key to training. Don't expect your cat to jump through hoops or roll over on command. However, you can expect your cat to stay within the boundaries of acceptable behavior in human society.

Emily Post for cats. It's probably best to make your training goal to cultivate good manners in your cat. Manners can be defined as performing normal and natural cat behaviors in the places, at the times, and in the way that satisfies both human and feline needs. This means finding the middle ground—in other words, what you can live with—and sticking to it. For example, it's unrealistic to think you can train your cat to never jump up on the dining room table. It's completely possible, however, to train him that it's bad manners to do so when humans are eating or when food is present.

Avoid bad habits. When it comes to behavior problems, most cat owners don't think in terms of prevention—and more's the pity. It may be cute when your 12-week-old kitten plays with your bare hand, but six months later when the now ten-pound beast sinks his full set of predator's teeth into your wrist, he's really only doing what he was taught to do. So, the best rule of thumb to follow is a common sense one: Never encourage any behavior you don't want to see later on, and always discourage any behavior you never want to see again.

Shape your cat's behavior. It's important to realize that certain cat behaviors can't be discouraged completely; they can only be shaped into a form that is socially acceptable in your household. This is also known as behavior modification.

A good example is scratching. This is an instinctive behavior for which many cats are declawed, lose their homes, or are even put to sleep each year. A better strategy is shaping the scratching behavior toward an acceptable object, such as a properly constructed scratching post, while simultaneously making other choices unpleasant or difficult. (For the complete regimen, see the section on scratching furniture in Chapter 8, "Common Behavioral Problems and Home Remedies.")

Accentuate the positive. The most successful, long-lasting, humane, and commonsense way to train or shape the behavior of any animal is positive reinforcement. The opposite method, negative reinforcement, punishes the animal for exhibiting a particular behavior in any way other than what the owner or trainer wants. In the example of scratching furniture, this would mean following the cat around the house 24 hours a day and correcting him every time he lays claw to upholstery. Since scratching is instinctive and can't be stopped, this method is doomed to failure anyway. Instead, the remedy offered in Chapter 8 calls for structuring the environment so that a correctly designed scratching post is always the best—and in some cases, the only—choice for scratching. Also, praising and petting the cat when he uses the post and offering minor corrections (not punishments) when he's caught in the act of scratching elsewhere will help modify the behavior.

NOW YOU'RE READY TO MOVE ON

The information in this chapter is a little academic, to be sure. But without it, none of the remedies in the next chapter will make complete sense. Remedying behavior problems can't be done by "cookbook" means. Every individual cat is unique, which means every individual cat's behavior is unique. Most likely, you'll have to adapt the remedies to fit your own cat's personality and the circumstances in your home. You're now armed with the basic tools you need to accomplish that.

> Towser, a Scottish cat, caught about 25,000 mice in her lifetime. At age 23, she was still catching three mice daily.

Behavior and Training

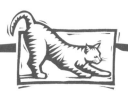

Common Behavioral Problems and Home Remedies

Is your cat turning your couch into confetti? Or your best carpet into a litter box? Maybe she's up on the table at mealtimes or dashing through doors and into trouble.

Next to allergies, behavior problems are probably the most common reason cats lose their homes. In fact, a lot of cat owners probably flipped right past everything else in this book and headed straight to the page with the behavior problem that's driving them crazy.

But before you go on, be sure you've read and digested Chapter 7, "Behavior and Training." Before you can tackle behavior problems, you need to know a little bit about cat behavior and what your cat is trying to tell you.

Biting and Scratching (humans and other cats)

You're walking down the hallway in your home, minding your own business, when suddenly your cat flings herself at your ankle, sinking in her teeth and claws, then dashes away. Is it an aggressive attack? An expression of jealousy? Possibly, but it might be neither.

A cat who bites or scratches when in pain, frightened, or being forced to do something she doesn't want to do doesn't have a behavior problem; she's acting like a normal cat. Problem biting and scratching is usually either a learned habit or miscommunication, both of which can be corrected over time. Sometimes, however, sudden unprovoked biting or scratching can be the result of a nervous system disorder or a serious disease. (Note: Any bite or scratch you get from a cat who does not have a current rabies vaccination should prompt a call to your own doctor; always assume cats have not had rabies shots unless they have a current rabies tag or registration.)

Who taught her the trick? Many kittens learn to use human limbs as toys, climbers, and scratching posts. Many owners are surprised to learn that they are the ones who taught their young cats these bad habits.

Here are some rules to follow:

- Never allow or encourage a kitten or cat to play with your bare hand or foot.

- Never think you can get around the first rule by wearing protective gloves. There should always be some sort of appropriate cat toy between your limbs and your cat's teeth and claws. A tiny kitten may look cute climbing your pant leg or batting at your thumb, but you'll be singing a different tune when she repeats those behaviors as a full-grown cat.

It's probably play. Pouncing, biting, and smacking are normal parts of cat play behavior. The only way your cat knows how to relate to you is as if you were another cat. It's up to you to explain to her—in ways she'll understand—that she's being too exuberant.

First, make sure your cat has enough outlets for normal feline play. Just leaving some toys around isn't enough; cats need active and interactive play. So play with her. Get her running, jumping, and batting at toys. If she tries to grab at you during a play session, grab her gently by the scruff of the neck, firmly (but not too loudly) say "No," and immediately substitute a proper cat toy for her to play with.

Boredom during the day may encourage your cat to be overly exuberant in playing with you, too. If you have a single cat, consider getting her a feline friend.

A break from the routine. Once your cat has the habit of playing with you by biting and scratching, just changing the rules probably won't be enough to get her to stop. Try to notice when she's most likely to chomp your hand or swat your ankle, then deliberately set up one of those situations. Have a spray bottle or squirt gun full of room temperature water handy, and give her a spritz the moment she digs in with tooth or claw. Don't yell at her or pursue her with the water; you want her to associate the action with the inconvenience of getting suddenly wet.

Defensive biting and scratching. Teeth and nails are a cat's primary weapons. If other warnings don't work, cats will bite and scratch to protect themselves. Pay attention to your cat's vocal and body language; she'll usually let you know when she's on the brink of defensive biting or scratching. You don't have to show a cat who's boss by forcing the issue once she's warned you. The best approach is to back off whatever it is she doesn't like or use a safe method of restraint, if it's something that must be done. (See the section on restraining a cat in Chapter 5, "At-Home Health Care: Practical Skills.")

Likewise, look for warning signals when a cat is aggressive with other cats. If your cat is warning another cat that she's ready to bite or scratch, do not try to touch or restrain either of them. The cats have their attention focused on each other, and the "fight or flight" response is in full readiness. Your touch can actually trigger a fight. Instead, try and distract both cats by stamping your foot, clapping your hands, and shouting "No!" in a sharp, loud tone.

Unprovoked aggression. Sudden, unprovoked, and vicious attacks are especially scary. This is not just a cat swatting at your ankles and perhaps causing a little scratch or running your hose. This is send-someone-to-the-emergency-room kind of stuff.

Sometimes, serious biting and scratching is the result of miscommunication: Something startles the cat, and she has the impression that the person or pet nearest her is responsible. Other times, however, there really is something physically wrong with the cat that causes her to actually attack without cause or warning. If your cat's bites and swats rarely break the skin, they're probably "inhibited" play bites and scratches. A cat who launches a serious attack (with multiple or deep bites, for example) should be carefully examined by a veterinarian.

☎ WHEN TO CALL THE VET

If your cat is launching serious attacks, especially without warning or provocation, get her in for a thorough veterinary exam as soon as possible. Cats often know when there's something going wrong with them but can't put it into words. The aggression might be a reaction to pain, a hormonal change, or the sign of a problem with her nervous system.

Chewing

Fortunately, cats don't have the strong need for chewing that dogs have. However, they are very prone to gnawing certain objects or materials, particularly telephone and electrical cords—a potentially fatal habit. Less dangerous but equally as annoying is the occasional cat who likes to gnaw the wood on the corners of furniture or chew paper or plastic.

Make it hard to swallow. There are several commercial products that can be applied to whatever the cat is chewing—especially wires and cords—to correct the behavior. Pet stores sell a variety of bitter pet repellents. Basically, these are just liquids that leave a bad-tasting residue when they dry. You might be able to accomplish the same thing by applying bitters to whatever the cat is munching on. Enclosing phone wires and electrical cords in hard conduiting or running them under rugs, inside walls, or along moldings may be better long-term solutions, though.

Give her what she wants. It's possible you have a cat who just likes to chew. Sometimes, a hard rubber chew toy or rawhide stick will satisfy the craving. Edible chewies for cats have been marketed from time to time but with only limited success.

Is she telling you something? Chewing can sometimes be a sign of boredom, tooth or mouth discomfort, or something missing from the cat's diet. Usually, though, the message from the cat is, "Don't leave any of this particular item laying around where I can reach it, unless you don't mind tooth holes in it."

When to Call the Vet

Chewing behavior rarely has a physical cause. However, your vet can help you determine a course of treatment or refer you to a competent behaviorist.

CLIMBING

Cats are natural vertical climbers and leapers. In other words, the higher a cat can go, the happier she often is. It's no big deal for a young, healthy cat to make a straight jump from the floor to a flat surface four or five feet off the ground. Panicked searches for "lost" cats frequently turn them up on top of refrigerators, on top of doors, or even inside cabinets that humans need a step stool to reach.

A cat's love of heights probably came about for security while sleeping. If you're at the highest vantage point, nobody can sneak up on you, and any other animal trying to climb up to get you has to use most of its legs and strength just to hang on.

Give her a place of her own. Build or buy one or more cat trees—a central post with perches and enclosed hiding places. You can use a large tree limb as the central post to give the piece a more natural look and make it more inviting for the cat. The base must be wide, sturdy, and well-weighted to prevent tipping over. The perches and hidey-holes are often carpeted to make them more comfortable and help blend in with decor or color schemes.

Make other options less appealing.
To discourage your cat from climbing or jumping on something, you need to make that action have a less pleasant outcome. Once again, you can set your cat up with the squirt gun or water bottle. Stake out the place in question, and spritz her once with room temperature water as soon as she makes her move. Using your voice to startle her off can work, too, but she may associate the correction with your presence, which is no help at all when you're not in the room.

This type of behavior usually doesn't require any veterinary attention. However, keep an eye on your cat in case she has a fall. While it's true most cats land on their feet, there are still risks of injury—especially internal injury—from the fall.

ESCAPING

Cat owners sometimes mistake those unexpected dashes for the door as the cat's way of expressing her need to be in the great outdoors. While the wide open spaces with all the interesting sights, smells, and sounds are certainly intriguing to cats, they will just as happily shoot through any forbidden door. It's largely a game, but if what's on the other side of the door is unsafe for the cat, it can be a deadly game.

Show her what's there. If your cat is intensely curious about what's beyond the door, get a leash and cat harness and take her out under controlled conditions. The fun part is usually getting past the door; once she's done that, the challenge is over, and she'll probably lose interest quickly.

Be sure nothing is driving her out. Cats may try and escape for the same reasons people do: There's something they want to get away from. A cat who's stressed—by the arrival of a new baby, the departure of an elderly companion cat, or the merciless teasing of a two- or four-legged member of the household—may simply want to get away from it all. Occasionally, there may be environmental stresses in your home that drive the cat out the door. One example was the family that got an ultrasonic home alarm system—silent to humans but well within a cat's range of hearing. The family would come home, deactivate the alarm, and open the door, and the cat, who'd been subjected to a constant barrage of ultrasonic noise all day, would streak out the door at a dead run.

Make it less fun. If your cat is door-dashing for the fun of it, you want to get the message across that it's no laughing matter. Load a water pistol or spray bottle with room temperature tap water and lure her into thinking you're going through the forbidden door. As soon as she makes a break for it, spritz her.

☎ WHEN TO CALL THE VET

Escape behavior usually doesn't require any veterinary attention.

FINICKY EATERS

Finickiness is one of the most famous of all feline traits. According to many behaviorists, however, it's a learned behavior and not an inborn one. Cats will happily eat the same food twice a day for their entire lives, provided it's nutritionally complete and tastes good enough.

Don't teach her the habit. Surprisingly, a lot of feline finickiness is taught to cats by their owners. Thinking the cat will get bored with a single flavor or brand, owners stock up on a variety of foods, trying different ones with each meal to determine a pet's favorites. If a cat walks away from a particular brand or flavor and the owner immediately opens another can, box, or bag, the cat quickly learns that finickiness pays. If you feel you must vary the flavors in your cat's diet, adopt the old-fashioned approach of, "Eat what's put in front of you. If you don't like it, you don't have to eat it—but that's all there's going to be until the next meal." Unless a cat eats absolutely nothing for a couple of meals running, there's no danger to her health if she has a few lean meals now and then.

Try the 20-minutes-and-up method. If you find yourself opening six cans at every meal and following your cat around the house, trying to coax her to have a nibble, you've got a serious finickiness problem going. At the next meal, put down a food you know the cat has eaten before. Wait 20 minutes, and then pick up the food and do

> Many people believe that all cats like fish, but no food is universally liked by cats.

not give any other food, snacks, or treats until the next meal. Repeat the process at that meal and every subsequent meal. Be prepared for an all-out tantrum by your cat—loud meowing, attempts to steal food, being an incredible pest, the works. Be strong and don't cheat to try to appease her. This method has a remarkable success rate. Many owners see improvement after three days, although some cats may persevere for several weeks.

☎ When to Call the Vet

If a previously good eater suddenly becomes finicky or finickiness persists despite the 20-minutes-and-up method, your cat may have a physical problem and need veterinary care. Any cat who quits eating completely or has a loss of appetite accompanied by other symptoms of illness should be seen by the veterinarian right away.

Knocking Things Down

Most of the time, cats send things crashing to the floor in the course of vigorous play; a wild run up the front hall culminates in a ricocheting leap from floor to couch to end table, sending the intervening lamp crashing to the floor in the process. Sometimes, though, a cat will deliberately nudge an item over the edge of a shelf or table, then gleefully dash away from the resulting chaos and infuriated humans.

Is it nature or nurture? "Toying" with prey is a common behavior in feline hunters. When your cat nudges a small, stationary object with her paw, she's practicing the same behavior. Your cat's instincts tell her that paperweight or knick-knack could turn out to be a mouse. Her poking paw would send it scurrying, giving her a good game (and possibly a good lunch).

However, once a cat learns that knocking something to the floor will bring humans on the double-quick, she may actually do it on purpose to get your attention, particularly if she feels that a meal is long overdue.

TALES FROM THE COUNTRY VET: MORRIS AND ME

I once got a call about the finickiest cat in the world, an orange tabby male called Morris. No, not *the* Morris, but one who was every bit as persnickety about his eating, and then some. Morris's owner insisted the only thing Morris would eat at all was tuna (a particularly expensive brand, packed in water—never the off-brands and never packed in oil) and chicken livers, panfried in a little olive oil. Now, it seemed, Morris was starting to turn his nose up at the liver, so what else, the owner wanted to know, could I suggest feeding him?

I told the owner to bring Morris in for an exam. He was a reasonably healthy cat, considering his limited diet of late. Everything else checked out normally, so I prescribed the 20-minutes-and-up method, using a good-quality, premium-brand dry food. After several false starts ("Well, yes...I did give him a few treats before I went to bed so he'd stop meowing so much."), Morris's owner finally stuck to his guns, and Morris learned to eat like a normal cat—although it took over four months to get there!

Give her something else to do. A bored cat will find her own ways to amuse herself and shoving things off high places to watch them drop is often one of them. Ample appropriate toys, climbing and hiding places to call her own, and a playmate—preferably another cat— can provide her with better options.

Take temptation out of her way. Low shelves, countertops, or tables lined with knick-knacks, collectibles, or small easel-backed picture frames are an invitation to disaster in a home with cats. Anything that won't survive a trip from whatever surface it's on to the floor should be put somewhere else or surrounded by a cat-proof barrier, such as putting porcelain figurines in a glass-front case rather than on open shelves.

☎ WHEN TO CALL THE VET

This type of behavior usually doesn't require any veterinary attention. However, keep an eye on your cat to make sure she doesn't knock anything down on top of herself.

LITTER BOX ACCIDENTS

Of all cat behavior problems, these are the ones owners complain about the most—and with good reason. Besides the mess and damage, inappropriate elimination is unsanitary and creates an unpleasant (and often malodorous) atmosphere in the home. Cats have an instinct to dig in loose materials and bury their urine and feces, and many of them adapt this instinct to the litter box with few problems. But it's still something they have to learn, and they often need help to get the lesson right.

Boxes, boxes everywhere. Litter boxes and litter should be the first things you buy when you decide to get a cat. Get them set up before the cat sets a single paw in your home. Make sure they are clean, easy to find, and numerous enough. Many cats dislike using a box that another cat has recently used (even if that other cat is herself), so the rule of thumb is: The number of litter boxes in the house should equal the number of cats in the house plus one. Thus, if you have two cats, you should have at least three litter boxes; even households with just one cat should have at least two boxes.

Keep it simple. Deodorizing litters, antibacterial litters, high-tech litters—all of these gimmicks used to sell various kinds of cat box fillers are aimed at the creatures that buy the litter, not necessarily the ones that use it. There's nothing wrong with using a litter that makes your job of tending to the litter box a little easier or a little less unpleasant, but some cats may be put off by the additives, perfumes, and chemical deodorizers used in some of these products. And that means they'll choose to do their business elsewhere. A plain cat box filler like ground clay (unscented) usually works fine.

Stop the madness. Once a cat starts eliminating outside of the litter box, do not assume she'll learn to use the box on her own. Cats habitually return to the same places to eliminate, a habit that's reinforced by the lingering odor of urine or feces. Since a cat's sense of smell is far superior to ours, cleaning up a litter box accident so that you can no longer detect the odor may not be enough to deter the cat from doing it again. Enzyme-based pet odor neutralizers actually break down the chemical structure of urine and feces residue so that your cat can no longer smell it. Pet supply stores usually carry at least one or two brands.

Block the favorite spots. Deny your cat access to places where she's eliminated outside the litter box. Physical barriers work well, but if that's not possible, try covering the spots with tinfoil or double-sided tape. This provides a barrier to the odor and a texture the cat won't want to walk on. If possible, consider placing a litter box directly on top of the inappropriate spot, and then gradually move the box an inch or so every few days, until it's where you want it to be.

Common Behavioral Problems and Home Remedies

Be your cat's personal trainer. When your cat first comes home, keep her in one room with a litter box. Once she's using that box consistently, give her the run of more rooms. Usually, this is enough to lock in the habit. However, a cat who doesn't completely get the hang of the litter box—or backslides and starts eliminating in other places—needs some additional training.

The best method is to use a large portable dog kennel. Set the cat up in the kennel with litter and water and give her meals in there, too. When you see her use the litter box, let her out for a recess. Keep an eye on her, and return her to her private quarters after an hour or two. The next time you see her use the litter box, let her out again. The idea is, she only gets free run of the house when she uses the litter box. This strategy can train (or retrain) a cat to use the litter box in as little as two or three weeks—but longer isn't uncommon, either.

What's the cause? A cat who suddenly begins eliminating in inappropriate places could be announcing that she doesn't feel well. You'll never make any progress on getting her to use the litter box consistently if there's a physical cause for the unwanted behavior, so get her to the vet as soon as possible.

Location, location, location. Sometimes, there's something about the location of the litter box the cat objects to. Maybe it's too far out of the way (down in a basement or up in an attic, for example) or too hard to get into or out of (especially for small kittens or elderly cats). Sometimes, air fresheners or other odors in the room will keep the cat away. Pine and citrus, for example, are pleasing smells to us but may be offensive to cats. Also, loud noises, such as a nearby stereo, may disturb your cat when she's doing her business.

☎ When to Call the Vet

Before you try to treat inappropriate elimination as a behavior problem, take your cat to the vet for a thorough exam. If your vet rules out a physical cause, you know it's probably a straight behavior problem. However, even if there is a physical problem and your vet treats it successfully, your cat still has developed the habit of eliminating someplace other than litter box; you'll still need to follow the steps for correcting the behavior problem.

Pica or Eating Nonfoods

Every kitten has tried to eat kitty litter—and many have succeeded. Far from being a behavior problem, this is part of a cat's natural curiosity, and one of the ways a growing kitten explores her world and learns about what counts as food—and what doesn't. Other cats, however, will get a yen for strange items that don't really qualify as food, some of which may even be unsafe.

Keep temptation out of her way. Rubber bands, paper clips, twist ties, bits of foil, and cellophane wrappers are some of the everyday things that cats love to explore with their mouths. Whether swallowed accidentally or on purpose, these otherwise harmless items can cause potentially deadly blockages in the cat's digestive system. Cat owners should be careful to keep tiny, easily swallowed items safely in drawers.

Is she telling you something? Pica is occasionally a signal that a cat isn't getting enough to eat—or enough of the right nutrients. It can also sometimes be a sign that something is out of balance in the cat's body. Other times, the cat gets into the habit of eating odd things out of boredom—in which case, more play or a playmate often takes care of the problem.

☎ When to Call the Vet

It's always a good idea to consult your vet if your cat develops a craving for a nonfood or if you know she's swallowed a potentially dangerous item like a rubber band.

Scratching
(on furniture and other things)

Every kind of cat, from lions and cheetahs to Siamese and alley cats, have an instinctive need to scratch. Scratching behavior serves three functions: marking territory, keeping the cat's claws in proper condition, and stretching the muscles and ligaments in the toes and feet. Declawing (the surgical removal of the first joint of the cat's toes, which includes both the nail and the cells from which new nails grow) does not stop scratching behavior, although it tends to reduce the amount of damage the cat can do. Your goal, then, is not to stop your cat from scratching—that can't be done—but rather to limit her scratching to the places you choose.

> Just as we like to stretch, a cat often has the urge to claw something after waking up.

Give her a good scratching post—or two, or three. Remember the three reasons for scratching, and get a post that meets all those needs. It should be tall enough for an adult cat to reach up and get a good stretch. It has to be sturdy enough that a 10- to 15-pound cat repeatedly pulling on it near the top won't bring it toppling over on her head. This would be a quick way to train her not to scratch on the post! The post should be covered with a nubby, coarsely woven fabric that shows scratching damage, such as sisal cloth. Cats are attracted to textured surfaces as scratching zones, and the coarse weave lets them hook in and get a good stretch. Being able to see the results of their handiwork reinforces the territory marking part of scratching. These are the absolute basic requirements for a proper scratching post.

Put it in plain sight. Remember the last time you were looking for a particular address and none of the houses were clearly marked? You probably muttered to yourself, "Why don't they mark these things so people can see them?" Your cat's scratching damage is how she marks her territory—her address, so to speak. If the scratching post can't be seen from cat height (about six or seven inches off the ground) and from many angles in the room, your cat is more likely to ignore it and make her statement on your couch or carpet.

Take temptation out of the way. Try to structure your cat's environment so that the scratching post is the most accessible and attractive thing to scratch on. If you're committed to a lifetime of having cats, it's probably better to outfit your home with washable area rugs and hardwood floors than wall-to-wall deep-pile carpeting in every room. Likewise, furniture upholstered with textured weaves and wicker are almost certain to sustain scratching damage; if you know you'll always have cats, pick another decorating scheme.

Of course, there is an old-fashioned, tried-and-true way to keep cats from scratching expensive draperies, furniture, and carpeting: Put those pieces in one room, shut the door, and allow the cat to roam only in the other rooms.

Pause for claws. Trim your cat's nails regularly to reduce her ability to inflict serious scratching damage. If you're squeamish or your cat is particularly uncooperative, you can have your vet or groomer do it for you. (See the section on clipping your cat's nails in Chapter 2, "Care and Maintenance.")

Hide the damage. If your cat has already done some scratching damage, block it from her view. This means putting stereo speakers on high shelves, covering afflicted pieces of furniture with a sheet, or removing items behind closed doors. The good thing about scratching damage in inappropriate places is your cat has identified the locations she thinks are best for scratching. Once you cover or remove the damaged items, put a proper scratching post next to it or in its place.

Make some corrections, but accentuate the positive. Employ the spray bottle or squirt gun to correct occasional scratching in undesirable locations. Use positive reinforcement techniques to encourage your cat to use the scratching post exclusively: Dangle some toys from the top and encourage her to climb the post or bat at them; scrabble your fingertips on the fabric of the post to get her to start scratching there; physically remove her from scratching in an inappropriate spot and place her paws in scratching position where you want her to go. In all cases, lavish her with praises and petting for doing the right thing.

WHEN TO CALL THE VET

Scratching behavior rarely has a physical cause. However, your vet can help you determine a course of treatment or refer you to a competent behaviorist.

SHYNESS

More than just the fabled feline aloofness, shy cats can be all but invisible, running and hiding even from their owners. At some time during the day, virtually every cat wants to be alone and will find a secluded place to crawl into. But shy ones and "scaredy-cats" may spend most of their time out of sight. A cat that spends most of her time under the bed isn't having a good time—and may not be getting enough food, water, or exercise.

Why are some cats so shy? Some breeds are more reserved than others, and some cats, usually those who have not been socialized to humans, tend to be people-shy. In certain cases, the cat may be frightened of certain types of people—children or men, for example.

They only come out at night. Cats are naturally nocturnal animals. If your cat rarely comes out during the day, don't assume she's not prowling around the house at night. Since cats can have very quiet footfalls when they want to, you may not hear her—and you won't see her because you're asleep. By the way, just because you find her in the same hiding place in the morning that you left her in the night before also doesn't mean she spent the whole night there!

> The introverted type of behavior is usually established in the first weeks of life and typically develops when the kitten lacks social contact.

To try and help a shy cat feel more secure, try waiting until nightfall. Turn off all the lights and pull the shades. Then, wait and see if your scaredy-cat is more willing to venture out.

Try a little tenderness. Give a shy cat attention but on her own terms. Talk to her in her hiding place—perhaps even feed her there if she doesn't come out to eat. Give her space, but reassure her with your words, tone of voice, and actions, and let her know you mean her no harm. Be patient. Making progress on socializing a shy cat can take weeks or months.

Make it worth her while. Treats, soft talk, and petting can help coax a nervous cat into society. If you find something she particularly likes—a specific food, a rub behind the ear, grooming with the slicker brush—reserve it to give her only on occasions of social interaction.

Don't force the issue. Let a shy cat build her confidence on her own timetable. If you try to drag her out of her safe spot and force attention on her, you may actually make her more shy—or risk being bitten or scratched. There's no law that says your cat must greet your visitors or play with the neighbor children. If she wants to be a recluse on social occasions, let her.

☏ WHEN TO CALL THE VET

If a previously friendly cat starts acting antisocial or hides a lot, she could be signaling the onset of illness. Notify your vet right away.

SPRAYING

A lot of the practical correction of this problem is covered in the section on litter box accidents in this chapter, and there's also a discussion about the physical causes in the section on spraying in Chapter 6, "Common Physical Problems and Home Remedies." However, since urine spraying is a specific—and not uncommon—cat behavior, it also warrants its own detailed entry here.

This type of behavior most often appears in unneutered young adult male cats, although any cat can display it. Spraying behavior is exhibited when the cat backs up to a vertical surface with his tail erect and squirts urine. He may tread with his hind feet, and there's a telltale jiggling of the tail. Cats will sometimes exhibit this behavior without spraying any urine. The main purpose of urine spraying seems to be marking territory.

Alter early. Typically, male cats who are neutered before they reach full maturity (usually by the age of six or seven months) are much less likely to begin spraying. Once an intact male cat starts spraying, the habit will be hard to break—even after he's neutered. Do not count on successfully correcting urine spraying if the cat is not neutered.

Lessen the stress. Spraying is sometimes a cat's way of saying there's too much going on. A common cause of stress-induced spraying is multiple-cat households. It's not necessarily that the cat doesn't like living with other cats, it may just be that he feels the territory isn't big enough to accommodate everybody's "personal space."

If you suspect spraying may be stress related, eliminate or reduce the sources of stress, if possible. Help him cope by making sure he gets enough attention and exercise. And be certain he has places to retreat to in your home where he can get away from it all, such as a high shelf with a comfortable blanket, a cat tree, or other piece of cat furniture.

Check it out. Except in the case of an unneutered young adult cat, if your cat suddenly begins spraying, it could be a sign of a urinary tract disease or other health problem. As with neutering, spraying that starts with a physical problem can't be corrected until the physical problem is put right.

☎ WHEN TO CALL THE VET

If your cat sprays even once, contact your vet. This isn't a behavior you want to continue, and if there's a physical reason—or it's time for a male kitten to be neutered—you want to get it taken care of before the behavior becomes a permanent habit.

WOOL SUCKING

There's nothing quite so incongruous as seeing a big old former street cat sitting on top of a pink sweater, blissfully kneading with her front paws and sucking away like a tiny kitten. Although called wool sucking, cats who display this type of behavior

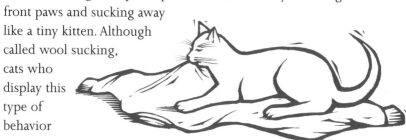

may go after other kinds of fabrics as well. At the very least, they can snag it, slobber on it, and shed hair all over it. But wool suckers are also prone to chewing and can destroy items such as expensive clothes, blankets, and comforters faster and more efficiently than moths or small children.

It's not completely clear why cats do it, although some behaviorists suspect it's more common in cats who were weaned too young. Certain breeds, most notably Siamese, are more prone to wool sucking, so it probably has a strong genetic factor.

If your cat is a wool sucker, don't despair; there are several guidelines you can follow in order to guard your garments from destruction.

Take temptation out of her way. It may be cute to see your cat all cuddled up in your sweater drawer, but if she turns out to be a wool sucker, you may end up having to replace your wardrobe. Get into the habit of putting clothing, blankets, towels, and other textiles away in securely closing drawers, closets, and cabinets.

Either way, it's fiber. Sometimes, a cat's desire to suck and chew fabric fibers can be curbed by giving her more dietary fiber. A crunchy dry food is higher in fiber than canned food and may provide the oral stimulation that a wool sucker craves. If your wool sucking cat shows an interest, you can also try tearing up a leaf or two of lettuce for her to munch on instead of your cardigan.

The old switcheroo. When you see your cat heading for your favorite wool sweater, replace the sweater with a chew toy or a wool-covered toy. Providing your cat with plenty of toys to chew on may prevent her from going for your expensive garments.

Age before beauty. As a preventative measure, before you get another pet, consider the cat's age. Since there might be a connection between early weaning and wool sucking, you may want to consider adopting kittens who are at least ten weeks old and have been with their mothers the whole time. Although weaning often occurs around five weeks of age, a ten-week-old kitten is sure to have made the transition completely.

WHEN TO CALL THE VET

Wool sucking usually doesn't require any veterinary attention. However, keep an eye on your cat to make sure she doesn't swallow any loose strings; this can cause intestinal problems, which require immediate attention.

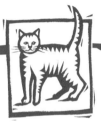

Where to Learn More

As good as this book is, it's not the last word. There are lots of knowledgeable people and fine organizations out there to help you along the way.

Need to find a veterinarian or a veterinary specialist? Contact the American Veterinary Medical Association or the American Animal Hospital Association. Wonder what's being done to protect cats and other animals? Talk to the Humane Society of the United States or the American Humane Association. Curious about breeders and cat shows? There are several breed associations listed here. There are even a few interesting World Wide Web sites for you to check out.

Good luck—and enjoy your cat!

ALTERNATIVE VETERINARY MEDICINE

American Holistic Veterinary Medical Association
2214 Old Emmorton Road
Bel Air, MD 21015
(410) 569-0795
Web site: http://www.altvetmed.com

American Veterinary Chiropractic Association
623 Main Street
Hillsdale, IL 61257
(309) 658-2920
E-mail: AmVetChiro@aol.com

National Center for Homeopathy
801 North Fairfax Street, Suite 306
Alexandria, VA 22314
(703) 548-7790
Web site: http://homeopathic.org

International Veterinary Acupuncture Society
PO Box 2074
Nedorlund, CO 80466
(303) 258-3767

 ## ANIMAL HOSPITALS, VETERINARIANS & FELINE SPECIALISTS

American Animal Hospital Association
PO Box 150899
Lakewood, CO 80215-0899
(303) 986-2800

American Association of Feline Practioners
    and the Academy of Feline Medicine
6808 Academy Parkway NE
Suite B-1
Albuquerque, NM 87109
(505) 343-0088

American Veterinary Medical Association
1931 North Meacham Road, Suite 100
Schaumburg, IL 60173-4380
(847) 925-8070 or 1-800-248-AVMA
Web site: http://www.avma.org
E-mail: 73711.555@compuserve.com

Cornell Feline Health Center
College of Veterinary Medicine
Cornell University
S3113 Sherman Hall
Ithaca, NY 14853
(607) 253-3414

 ANIMAL PROTECTION

American Humane Association
63 Inverness Drive East
Englewood, CO 80112-5117
(303) 792-9900

The Humane Society of the United States
2100 L Street NW
Washington, DC 20037
(202) 452-1100
Web site: http://www.hsus.org

Where to Learn More

Cat Breed & Show Associations

American Cat Association, Inc. (ACA)
8101 Katherine Avenue
Panorama City, CA 91402
(818) 781-5656

American Cat Fanciers Association (ACFA)
PO Box 203
Point Lookout, MO 65726
(417) 334-5430
Web site: http://www.acfacat.com/.

The Cat Fanciers Association, Inc. (CFA)
PO Box 1005
Manasquan, NJ 08736-0805
(908) 528-9797
Web site: http://www.cfainc.org/cfa/.

Cat Fanciers Federation, Inc. (CFF)
PO Box 661
Gratis, OH 45330
(513) 787-9009

The International Cat Association (TICA)
PO Box 2684
Harlingen, TX 78551
(210) 428-8046
Web site: http://www.tica.org/

Pet Loss Support Hotlines

California
University of California-Davis
School of Veterinary Medicine
Davis, CA 95616
(916) 752-4200
(916) 752-3602 to order free brochures
☉ Hours: 6:30 P.M. to 9:30 P.M., Pacific time, Monday through Friday.

Florida
University of Florida
College of Veterinary Medicine
Box 100124
Gainesville, FL 32610
(352) 392-4700; then dial 1 and 4080
☉ Hours: 7 P.M. to 9 P.M., Eastern time, Monday through Friday.

Illinois
Chicago Veterinary Medical Association
Riser Animal Hospital
5335 West Touhy
Skokie, IL 60077
(630) 603-3994
☉ Hours: 7 P.M. to 9 P.M., Central time, Monday through Friday.

Massachusetts
Tufts University School of Veterinary Medicine
200 Westboro Road
North Grafton, MA 01536
(508) 839-7966
☉ Hours: 6 P.M. to 9 P.M., Eastern time, Monday through Friday.

MICHIGAN

Michigan State University
College of Veterinary Medicine
A135 East Fee Hall
East Lansing, MI 48824
(517) 432-2696
☺ Hours: 6:30 P.M. to 9:30 P.M., Eastern time,
Tuesday through Thursday.

OHIO

Ohio State University
College of Veterinary Medicine
101 Sisson Hall
1990 Coffey Road
Columbus, OH 43210
(614) 292-1823
☺ Hours: 6:30 P.M. to 9:30 P.M., Eastern time,
Monday, Wednesday, Friday.

VIRGINIA

Virginia-Maryland Regional College of Veterinary Medicine
The Veterinary Teaching Hospital
Duck Pond Drive
Blacksburg, VA 24061
(540) 231-8038
☺ Hours: 6 P.M. to 9 P.M., Eastern time, Tuesday and Thursday.

WORLD WIDE WEB SITES

American Board of Veterinary Practitioners
http://www.psln.com/medhead/abvp.html
Canine and feline specialists, focusing on "whole patient" concept of practice.

American Holistic
Veterinary Medical Association Directory
http://www.altvetmed.com/associat.html
Directory of holistic veterinarians and related articles.

American Veterinary Medical Association
http://www.avma.org/home.html
Information and links for veterinarians and pet owners.

Myths and Facts About Cats
http://www.cfainc.org/cfa/articles/myths-facts.html
Informative articles from Cat Fancy Association, Inc.

NetVet and The E-Zoo
http://netvet.wustl.edu
Award-winning website; lots of information and links.

Where to Learn More

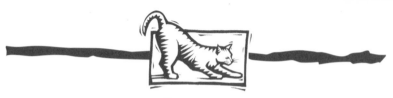

INDEX

Index

Index